FORESKIN

Foreskin

A CLOSER LOOK

An expanded, updated edition of *Foreskin*

by Bud Berkeley
with illustrations by Peter Leko

Boston ♦ Alyson Publications, Inc.

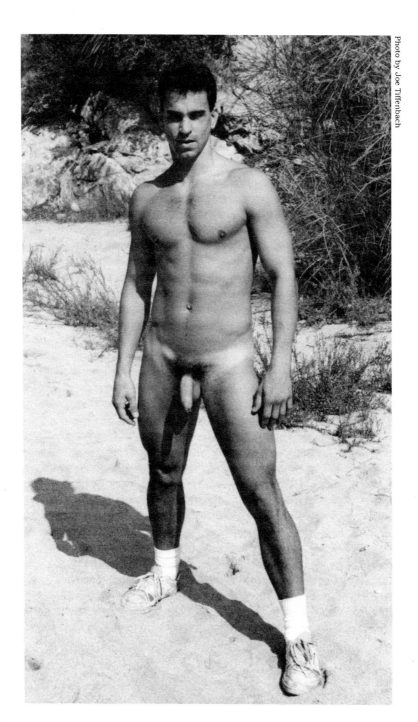

Typeset and printed in the United States of America.

This is a trade paperback from Alyson Publications, Inc.,
40 Plympton St., Boston, Mass. 02118.
Distributed in the U.K. by GMP Publishers,
P.O. Box 247, London N17 9QR, England.

This book is printed on acid-free, recycled paper.

First Alyson edition: July 1993

5 4 3 2 1

ISBN 1-55583-212-1

Library of Congress Cataloging-in-Publication Data
Berkeley, Bud.
    Foreskin : a closer look / by Bud Berkeley ; with illustrations by
Peter Leko. — 1st Alyson ed.
        p.   cm.
    "An expanded, updated ed. of: Foreskin."
    ISBN 1-55583-212-1 (acid-free paper) : $9.95
    1. Circumcision.   I. Title.
GT2470.B47 1993
392'.1—dc20   93-10531
                                                                    CIP

CONTENTS

A note on the second edition 7

PART 1:

A TRAVELER ... UNCIRCUMCISED 11

1. Uncircumcised in Hollywood 13
2. Uncircumcised Abroad 22
3. Moslems and Christians 29
4. In the Shadow of the Pyramids 36
5. The Uncircumcised Society of America 43

PART 2:

A LONG HISTORY OF THE AMERICAN FORESKIN 47

1. The British Empire Meets the Sword of Islam 51
2. Casualties of War 75
3. Our Search for the "Natural" 87

PART 3:

DEAR BUD: CIRCUMCISED AND UNCIRCUMCISED 103

1. Stretching It, Smelling It, Loving It 107
2. Options, Opinions 140
3. Icons, Numbers, Choices 175

A NOTE ON THE SECOND EDITION

The original edition of *Foreskin* was well received by both readers and critics. For several months it appeared on the best-seller list at A Different Light bookstores in Los Angeles and New York. In New Zealand, customs officials seized the book and presented it to the Indecent Publications Tribunal. According to an Auckland newspaper article, "Judge R.R. Kearney, chairman of the tribunal, found that [*Foreskin*] contained considerable research devoted to the historical and social attitudes to the uncircumcised male." He ruled that "the publication has very limited appeal. It does contain some material harmful to younger readers and the Tribunal accordingly classifies it as indecent in the hands of persons under the age of 16." *Foreskin* was thus allowed into New Zealand and soon thereafter one Auckland book dealer wrote, "The book is selling like hotcakes!"

I wrote *Foreskin* primarily for members of the Uncircumcised Society of America (USA), from whom much of the material was collected. It was first published in 1983, and has had three printings during the past decade.

A review of the first edition made me realize that I had succeeded in at least one of my goals. Book reviewer John Erickson wrote in the August 10, 1983, edition of the Los Angeles *Edge*,

> One of the first promises I made when I took over this column was that I would, at all cost, avoid the use of "I" and the phrases, "In my opinion" and "I think." ... When I was handed the book [*Foreskin*] to review my immediate thought was, "Oh no, *I* cannot be bothered with this when there was

so much more out there that needs *my* attention." Egos are amazing. What I said aloud was, "Oh Puh-leeze, does the world really need a book on foreskin?"

"My humblest apologies to my editor, to [the authors] and most certainly to the readers of this column," Erickson continued.

Plainly speaking, *Foreskin* sounds like another porno rag — which, through florid prose and redundant narratives, is generally nothing so much as a sophomoric attempt at titillation. *Foreskin* is not that. It is the first step in ... exploring the idea that erotic, social, religious and Oedipal urges contribute to man's proclivity toward male circumcision. The objectivity of the authors is most refreshing.

A second review claimed the history of circumcision in the first edition to be "well researched but breathless." Another claimed that, while the text was informative, the book had too many photos of penises to make it "legitimate."

For this second edition of *Foreskin*, I went back to my bibliography for a more in-depth look at the history of circumcision, and to review the increased awareness in the past decade of both the benefits and risks of circumcision, as well as of the natural values of the foreskin. The anti-circumcision movement has grown into a powerful advocacy machine but, in the meantime, AIDS and other important medical issues have highlighted the complexity of the issue. In this new edition I have tried to provide an overview of recent progress, but without seeming quite so "breathless."

I first wrote about my own personal experiences with foreskin in *Blueboy*, under the title, "How I Became President of the USA." It generated a great deal of interest in the subject of foreskin and circumcision, and I got many letters from men revealing experiences similar to my own. For this new edition of *Foreskin*, I have, reluctantly, decided to reveal more of my lifetime involvement with the subject matter.

I want to acknowledge historian Allen Edwardes, whose bibliographies were used extensively in this edition of *Foreskin*. Most unfortunately, his wonderful books (*The Jewel in the Lotus, The Rape of India, Death Rides a Camel,* and *Erotic Judaica,* all published by Julian Press from 1959 through 1967) are now out of print. Marilyn Milos, director of the

National Organization of Circumcision Resource Centers, allowed me to quote from her informative *N.O.C.I.R.C. Newsletter.* Dr. Aaron Fink, M.D., kept me informed of his efforts in the AIDS problem. I want to thank my friend and colleague, Egyptologist and circumcision historian Alfred V. Hodenschwingh, for allowing me to quote freely from his excellent work, *Circumcision in Ancient Egypt.* My most heartfelt thanks goes to the hundreds of members of the USA, whose loyalty and continued generosity in the sharing of their researched material, as well as of their personal experiences, has contributed greatly to the completion of this second edition.

WARNING

No statements, opinions, or other information contained in this book should be construed in any way as medical advice. Some passages are quoted from licensed medical professionals and they are so indicated. Many passages represent correspondence from members of the Uncircumcised Society of America which must be accepted as personal experience and not medical opinion. For medical advice, please consult your physician.

PART 1

A TRAVELER ...
UNCIRCUMCISED

"Foreskins fascinate me!" said my handsome young French visitor as he fingered his elegantly con-toured penis. "I suppose it's because I don't have one of my own," he continued. I was surprised; French boys aren't circumcised! Then he explained: "It happened in Paris, when I was nine years old. The school doctor decided my foreskin was too tight so he cut it off. After-ward, the other boys treated me as if I was ... how you say it? ... a circus freak. They pulled down my pants and laughed. Other Parisian boys all had their foreskins. I felt so ashamed of my penis."

Philippe continued as the neatly wrinkled skin just behind the bare glans of his circumcised cock began to smooth out, "I came to California last year to attend the university and I was very surprised to see so many circum-cised penises in the gymnasium showers. My penis was not a stranger there. I was no longer ashamed. But now I have a strange desire of which my girlfriend would fail to understand. I would like an uncircumcised man to stretch his foreskin over my naked penis." Philippe's penile skin was now stretched smoothly over a long, stiffening shaft as he eyed my foreskin. "Do you think it's possible for you to..." Hey, Philippe, is that what you want? Fine, let's do it! *"Oh, monsieur, mais oui..."*

"How does it happen that you, being an American, are not circumcised?" Philippe panted. "Why did you start writing about foreskins? Start researching circumcision history? Organize the Uncircumcised Society of America?"

Relax, my sexy Parisian, and I'll tell you all about it...

1. Uncircumcised in Hollywood

*F*oreskins were hard to find in Hollywood when I was growing up there. In fact, nobody except me had one. My two brothers, my cousins, my early playmates, and all the cadets at the boys' school had long since been circumcised.

My parents worked in the motion picture industry, and when I was born it was "in" for their set to give birth at the Hollywood Hospital. I don't know how my foreskin got out of that place alive. Everyone I knew in my childhood had been born there and not a vestige of prepuce could be found among them. I suspect that my father had something to do with it. I was his firstborn, his namesake, and as he too was uncircumcised, he left me uncut as well. He didn't do me a favor ... I hated my foreskin.

I was about five years old when I started attending a boys' school affiliated with the military school next door. On the very first day we were forced to take showers; I lined up, naked, alongside the boys with whom I was to spend my future school years. I'm sure we eyed each other with a healthy curiosity ... but to my horror they pointed at my penis and laughed. My fellow cadets never allowed me to forget that experience. As we reached puberty and experimented together, I was constantly teased about my uncircumcised dick. In the showers with visiting athletic teams my cock got yanked and as everyone turned to see what was going on, someone would yell, "When are they going to trim your tail, Berkeley?" I wanted to have a penis just like all the others. I wasn't about to admit it, though, to those brats.

On weekends I went home, where my brothers and I lived a confining boyhood. We were never allowed to leave the acreage surrounding our huge old house except for trips to the candy store with Warren, our chauffeur. We loved old Warren. Occasionally my parents gave big barbecues for their Hollywood friends and Warren donned a tall chef's cap and boiled the crawdads. Those parties provided the only excitement any of us had around home. Lots of movie stars got drunk and jumped in the pool. We laughed. We were happy because our parents were around on those weekends. Otherwise, we were alone with Warren, his wife May, and sometimes our Quaker grandmother, who thought my parents were going to hell with their riotous living.

One evening as I sat at the top of the staircase, a neighbor came by, carrying a small white baby pig under her arm. "Here, you can play with Geronimo," she said to me. My grandmother suddenly rushed from her room and screeched, "Don't touch that filthy thing!" I ignored her, and picked up Geronimo and caressed him. My grandmother didn't speak to me for a week. "Aren't you ashamed not minding me, young man?" she finally blurted out.

"No! Geronimo wasn't filthy. He was clean," I yelled back at her.

"Well, he was probably cleaner than you are," she retorted. "I'm going to have your father look at you and if you are not skinning back and cleaning yourself down there we're going to have you cut back like your brothers." I took her threat of circumcision as a punishment for not behaving, as she meant it to be.

In later years I learned to appreciate many aspects of my grandmother's Quaker religion, and grew less fond of my dad's atheism. But her attitude toward my foreskin left its mark on me. She once threatened to have me "cut back" when she suspected me of masturbating: "It will lead you into sin and sickness!" she roared. Statements like that made me defiantly self-defensive about not being circumcised.

14

✦ ✦ ✦

"Push your skin back!" ordered the young doctor. Dissatisfied with my hesitation, he reached down and pushed my foreskin back and forth himself. My penis quickly stood at attention, and I turned red with embarrassment. The doctor came to the school monthly to give each cadet a physical exam. I was fourteen and I learned to dread the moment I would be called out of class for my turn. Each month he watched my foreskin slide back and forth and my dick get stiff. Then, he would quietly write out a note, seal it, and tell me to give it to my parents. Intuitively, I knew those notes concerned circumcision. I hid them.

I was much too traumatized by the thought of circumcision to discuss it, especially with my parents. One day my grandmother found the hidden notes and gave them to my father. They argued, but I hid and didn't hear what they were saying. A few days later it was my mother who took me to the office of our family doctor. He quickly looked over my penis and asked me right out, "Do you want all that extra skin removed?"

"No!" I shouted. I wasn't about to return to school with a trimmed tail and let those brats have a laugh on me. Doc said that my foreskin was nice and loose and if I washed it out every day I could keep it. That was that.

When it was time to again go the school doctor, he set me on my lifelong path of researching the history and practice of circumcision. Pushing my foreskin tightly back on my boner to make my penis look circumcised, the doctor said, "See, doesn't that look better? Don't you think streamlined dicks look better, Berkeley? Don't you want a handsome dick like Joe Scott's?" Joe was the best football player in the school. Although I was the best competitive swimmer, I admired football players and Joe was my hero.

I said, "All football players aren't circumcised. My dad was a football player and he's got one just like mine."

The doctor answered, "But your dad comes from an earlier generation. Today, all boys are streamlined like Joe Scott, and you know very well that you're the only cadet in this school who hasn't been streamlined. Wouldn't you like me to circumcise it so that you'll look just like Joe?" I stood there with a full erection while I pondered his proposition. He really seemed to want to cut me back and I didn't want to disappoint him. Besides, I was taught that adults, especially doctors, were always right. Suddenly I felt a strange attraction to this man. I liked having his hand on my penis — and the feeling frightened me. I pulled my penis out of his grip and grabbed my clothes. I guess I startled him and his face flushed. He told me to think about getting circumcised and that he expected my decision the following month.

I thought about it all right! Alone in my bed at night I thought about the doctor, about how good-looking he was, about circumcision, about him circumcising me, about how my penis would look after it was circumcised, how it would feel, about Joe Scott's great-looking dick ... and about those other damned cadets who would never let me live it down if the doctor trimmed my tail. The whole situation soon got intertwined with my sexual fantasies. I couldn't think of anything else. What the hell was circumcision all about, anyway? Why was I allowed to remain uncircumcised? Where did the whole thing start? Why did it start? Why should people care about my dick? Does it work better when circumcised? It is easier to aim? I searched at the school library for references to circumcision. Usually, all I could find was a definition, but even that fascinated me. I got erections by reading the definitions. It became an obsession. It was my secret interest.

Emory suddenly showed up at school. New cadets rarely enrolled midsession, but his father was important. New cadets were not easily accepted by the other guys, however, and Emory didn't quite fit in with our crowd. After all, most of us had lived together since we were little kids. We knew all about each other ... we had become so intimate we knew exactly when each cadet reached manhood and how far he could shoot. We were a true brotherhood.

Emory wasn't even a good athlete. I sort of felt sorry for him, standing around the swimming pool by himself. After the water polo game we headed for the showers and I happened to glance at Emory. I couldn't believe my eyes. He was uncircumcised. It was the first uncut cock I had seen on someone my age. I stared! I wasn't the only one staring. Everyone in the shower room had stopped to look at Emory's dick. These same fellows had pointed and laughed at my dick years earlier, but they stared in silence at Emory.

There was something strange about Emory's cock, however, besides being uncircumcised. His foreskin only half covered his glans. Maybe that was why everyone stared in silence. The only foreskin the school had seen was mine, which tapered off for a full inch in front of my cockhead. I think everyone was trying to figure him out: was he or was he not clipped? I was elated. Finally, I had a kindred cadet at school. Half a foreskin was better than none.

Emory rose and left the class when it was his turn to visit the school doctor. It was his first time, and my mind filled with speculation. Maybe he'll circumcise Emory and forget about me! I still hadn't decided what to say to the doctor. I didn't want to loose my foreskin, but I had a fascination about this doctor circumcising me. I fantasized that he would circumcise both Emory and me together. That would be fun. I tried to put the thought out of my mind, but it was hard to focus on schoolwork. Then my turn came to visit the doctor.

I took off my clothes and the doctor didn't touch my penis. He didn't even look at it. He seemed angry, unfriendly, and I was quickly dismissed. What did I do wrong? I felt guilty. He didn't even want to circumcise me anymore. Had I been right? Was the doctor going to trim Emory's tail instead of mine? I felt jealous. Hell, I had more foreskin than Emory; I had more to cut off. Why didn't he want to do it to me? That night I decided, "I'll show him. I'm not ever going to let anyone streamline me. I'm an old-fashioned uncircumcised boy and I'm going to stay that way."

I avoided Emory for several weeks, I suppose out of jealousy, but I took every opportunity to look at his dick to see what the doctor had done. It remained the same. "Halfmast" is what the fellows called it. Finally, I found us alone together, and I couldn't wait to ask him, "Did the doctor want to do something to your dick?"

He looked surprised and said, "Yes, he wanted to look at it. I pushed back my foreskin for him. Why?" I was embarrassed and said I was just kidding. Then he asked, "Why do all the guys stare at me in the showers?"

"I guess no one can figure out if your dick has been clipped or not," I answered frankly.

"Yeah? Well you can tell them I'm uncircumcised and I wouldn't want to be mutilated like them," he angrily retorted.

"Mutilated?" That took me by surprise. I was dumbfounded by the idea that circumcision was mutilation. Realizing that he, too, felt strongly about being uncircumcised, I told him, "Until you came along I was the only uncircumcised cadet in this school."

"Yeah," he said, "I noticed." He seemed bitter and I was about to walk away when he said something very soothing to me. "You're lucky, Berkeley, to have such a long foreskin. I'll bet it stays over your cock even when you have a boner. I'd like to see it."

For the first time I was proud of my foreskin. For the first time I had an uncircumcised friend with whom I could confide. Needless to say, we started comparing notes and foreskins. We spent hours together in the library reading about circumcision. We dug through the art books and studied photos of Greek statues.

Emory had a love-hate fascination with circumcision. Like me, just reading its definition gave him an erection. Yet he sneered at the circumcised cocks of our fellow cadets and called them "deadheads." We loved reading about Sir Richard Burton, the nineteenth-century explorer who translated *The Arabian Nights* and "found the practice of circumcision, and the great variety of ways in which the operation was performed, of absorbing interest."[1] We also found an ancient poem from the first-century Roman poet Marcus Matrialis, which gave us a private laugh:

> You do not stiffen, Maevus, except in sleep;
> And to keep yourself from pissing on your feet,
> You take clipt cock in hand; your fingers press
> and pump that shriveled, drooping shaft; and yet
> the most forceful jerks won't lift its dead head.
> Whose miserable cunt and butt does it vainly irritate?
> In any case, that shaft must thrive on some old bitch!

We had fun over that one and privately pointed at the "dead heads" in the school showers and snickered. We turned the tables on the clipcocks.

The cadets noticed that Emory and I had become close friends. He was still an outsider to them. They joked about our "baby dicks," and we occasionally heard the word "queer." It was usually aimed at Emory and not me, because, after all, I was one of them. Besides, I was the champion swimmer in the school. It was unfair because we didn't do anything together that the other guys weren't doing. We were mostly reading books. Finally, an unhappy Emory left the school and was soon forgotten by everyone except for me. I missed having an uncircumcised friend. I missed our evenings at the library. But I found myself being more involved with the activity I loved most: swimming.

As we entered our midteens, other cadets continued to tease me: "When are they going to make a man of you, Berkeley?" It was good-natured teasing, however, without any real sting. I liked the attention, especially as it was aimed at my cock.

I had grown bored with that damned boys' school, with the cadets I had known all my life, and with the closed society that seemed to be my birthright. I wanted out. I begged my father to let me spend my senior year at a public high school. My grandmother had died, my beloved May and Warren had left our service, and my father was shacking up with a starlet somewhere in the Hollywood Hills. He finally allowed my brothers and me to live with his sister in Beverly Hills and I enrolled at North Hollywood High School.

I was finally attending a coeducational public school, and I soon had a sweetheart. She was a beautiful redhead. My aunt didn't approve of redheads. She was from Seattle and raised by grandparents. My aunt decided that she was a bastard. She had come to Hollywood, where she lived with relatives, with the dream of becoming an actress. My aunt decided that she was only after my family connections. Unfortunately, my aunt was right about that. When my sweetheart was introduced to my father, she practically jumped into bed with him.

◆ ◆ ◆

"Appointment for circumcision," the nurse at the university hospital wrote next to my name. I had just arrived on the campus in Northern California, away from Hollywood for the first time. I didn't know a soul there. Now was my chance to get the trimming that I had decided I wanted. I was new in town, and no one would know that anything had changed.

However, I had to wait a few weeks for my turn with the campus circumciser and, during that time, I joined the swim team and pledged a fraternity. By the time my circumcision date arrived I was already in training. Still embarrassed by the subject, I just couldn't get myself to tell the coach why I needed to spend a few days out of the swimming pool. Besides, the fellows at the fraternity had already seen my dick and I knew that my long foreskin had been noticed. It was too late for a covert clipping. However, to my great surprise, I had noted that about half of my fraternity brothers also had foreskins dangling between their legs. For the first time in my life, I was not alone.

For two years I focused on writing for the campus newspaper, studying journalism and Egyptology, and other interests. I was too busy to give any further thought to circumcision. That interlude did not last. I had joined ROTC, and quickly rose in rank. While I resented the time that ROTC demanded, it kept me in school and out of the Army. Things were heating up in Asia and I was concerned about my college deferment.

One day, during my third year in college, the ROTC major called six of us aside and showed us a gruesome Army film about VD and hygiene. "You are the only uncircumcised officers under my command," he told us. "I have made arrangements for your circumcisions." As the six of us sat there, stunned, he passed out medical releases to sign.

Was I to be haunted by the threat of circumcision all my life? I was furious! Just who did this puny little major think he was, anyway? I still hadn't resolved the circumcision question in my own mind, but I wasn't going to allow this military punk to make the decision for me. I made the excuse that the varsity swim team had an important meet coming up and they needed me. The major said he'd talk to my coach and, this time, I told my coach everything. He called the major an asshole, put his arm around me, and said, "Son, I'll get you out of it. By the way, Berkeley, I'm also uncircumcised. Guys like us have to stick together. Right?" His words took a huge burden off my shoulders. The thought of uncircumcised men being a brotherhood, sticking together, haunted me for years to come.

Jim sat next to me in the ROTC officers' class. He was a handsome blond fellow who had made sexual overtures toward me. I ignored him, playing dumb, because he belonged to a rival fraternity. I liked the guy and was attracted to him, but fraternity rivals just didn't socialize. Rules were rules. He whispered to me, "Want to see my Army clip job?" I was horrified. He had been one of the six students called into the major's office with me. I hadn't known that any of the guys ended up on the circumcision bench. I laughed off his offer and quickly changed the subject. But secretly I longed to inspect Jim's newly circumcised penis.

After a swim training session I ran into Leon in the showers. Leon was the scion of a Napa wine country family: a tall, well-built, patrician-looking Italian youth. I had always admired his well-shaped body, especially his fine, sturdy penis, which had a foreskin as long as my own. Just looking at him made me feel good about myself. This time, I was shocked at what I saw. His foreskin had been sliced off, at the direction of that self-important little major, and his penis was ringed by a crooked, glaring red scar. His unveiled glans looked irritated and it flared out as if permanently swollen. That could have been *my* penis!

Leon's newly carved penis shocked me. He turned to hide his cock from view. I felt sorry for him and pretended not to have seen it. We discussed an upcoming football game, the weather, and the war in Asia. After that episode, I didn't want to know who else among my fellow young officers got the knife. I just felt lucky and kept my mouth shut. All those years of flirting with the idea of getting clipped suddenly changed. I didn't want to end up with a pecker that looked like Leon's. I left college intact.

NOTES

1. This observation was made by Edward Leigh, who edited Burton's book *The Erotic Traveler* (New York: G.P. Putnam's Sons, 1966).

2. Uncircumcised Abroad

*L*ondon was full of foreskins and, when I went to live there after college, I felt right at home. The navy had turned me down because I had a slight stutter. Stuttering ran in my family, and I always attributed it to our English lineage. After all, King George VI had been a stutterer. I didn't miss the military; I figured that once the navy got its hands on my foreskin it would have been history. So, instead of a military career, I ended up in the land of my ancestors.

I couldn't wait to look up the works of Sir Richard Burton in the British Museum. He was my hero. In his books, and in those of other geographers and anthropologists from his era, I found a treasure trove of exotic sexual lore. At last, here were books that offered more than definitions. My hours in the museum reading room gave me a much wider perspective on the entire subject of circumcision.

Early during my stay in London I found a swimming pool in the old Tottenham Court YMCA, and I spent hours swimming laps to stay in shape. As I showered after my workout one day, I noticed a clean-cut fellow next to me. Bouncing in front of him was an American-style clipcock — the first one I'd seen there for months. I was homesick for America, so I struck up a conversation with him. To my surprise, I heard an Australian accent in reply, rather than the American accent I'd expected. But our personalities clicked and we became friends. Still embarrassed in front of circumcised men, I kept pushing my foreskin back whenever we were naked together. I must have still had an inferiority complex about it.

"Keep your bloody hands off your foreskin!" Andy blurted one day. "I want to see it hanging low. Why do you think I'm attracted to you? There aren't enough foreskins where I come from. I'm not interested in other circumcised men at all." What a revelation! I had figured that gay men didn't like uncircumcised penises and I had no idea that a circumcised man would seek me out because of my foreskin.

Andy proceeded to educate me about erotic aspects of foreskin ownership that I'd never thought about. He stretched my foreskin as far as it would go, then slowly rolled it back over my glans and penile shaft so that the inner foreskin was stretched inside out, then he rolled it forward again ... in tantalizingly slow motion. Here was a fellow who knew more about my cock than I knew and he was circumcised. After several days of this I grew exhausted, but he wouldn't stop playing with my foreskin.

Andy was scheduled to leave England soon. As he prepared to depart he said, "If you go to Australia with me, I'll marry you."

"Marry a man?" I laughed.

"Well, I just want your cock," he smiled. "Can I take it home with me? I won't find one like that in Sydney. You've spoiled me." I flushed. As he said his good-bye, he surprised me with a long, passionate kiss. Only then did I realize how he felt about me. I thought about Andy in the months that followed. I played with my foreskin as if it was a new toy, and returned to my research with vigor.

✦ ✦ ✦

"I here propose to consider at some length this curious custom [circumcision]," Sir Richard Burton wrote in a footnote to "The Tale of the Damsel Tohfat Al 'Kulub'" in his translation of *The Arabian Nights*,

> which has prevailed among so many widely separated races. Its object has been noted ... to diminish the sensitivity of the glans, no longer lubricated with prostatic lymph; this part is hardened against injury and disease and its work in

coition is prolonged. On the other hand "the foreskin increases (the woman's) pleasure in sexual intercourse, and
therefore women prefer intercourse with uncircumcised
men rather than Turks," says Dimerbroeck (*Anatomie*). I
vehemently doubt the fact. Circumcision was doubtless
practiced from ages immemorial by the people of Central
Africa, and Welcker found traces of it in a mummy of the
sixteenth century B.C. The Jews borrowed it from the Egyptian priesthood and made it a manner of sacrament, "uncircumcised" being "unbaptized," that is, barbarian,
heretic. ... The simplest form of circumcision is mere amputation of the prepuce and I have noted the difference
between the Moslem and Jewish rite, the latter according
to some being supposed to heal in kindlier way.[1]

"The varieties of circumcision are immense," the nineteenth-century anthropologist continued in his notes.

Probably none is more terrible than that practiced in the
province of Al-Asír, the old Ophir, lying south of Al-Hijáz,
where it is called Salkh, lit. = scarification. The patient,
usually from ten to twelve years old, is placed upon raised
ground holding in right hand a spear, whose heel sets upon
his foot and whose point shows every tremor of the nerves.
The tribe stands about him to pass judgment on his for-
titude, and the barber performs the operation with the
Jumbiyak-dagger, sharp as a razor. First he makes a shal-
low cut, severing only the skin across the belly immediately
below the navel, and similar incisions down each groin; then
he tears off the epidermis from the cuts downwards and
flays the testicles and penis, ending with amputation of the
foreskin. Meanwhile, the spear must not tremble and in
some clans the lad holds the dagger over the back of the
stooping barber, crying "Cut and fear not!"[2]

In the museum, I found such an abundance of material
for my secret research that I buried myself there for months.
Burton continues,

The Bantu or Caffre tribes are circumcised between the ages
of fifteen and eighteen; the "Fetish Boys," as we called them,
are chalked white and wear only grass belts; they live
outside the villages in special houses under an old
"medicine-man," who teaches them not only the virile arts

24

but also to rob and fight. The "man-making" may last five months and ends in fetes and dances.[3]

How I wanted to follow in Burton's footsteps into Africa!

In London I met a handsome English actor who returned to America with me and became my "longtime companion." He was circumcised. But back in the U.S., circumcision, with all its traumas and insecurities, was soon forgotten. The good life in Northern California was too laid-back to worry about foreskin. Then I began traveling to Egypt ... and again my foreskin became an object of contention.

✦ ✦ ✦

"Americans beeg," said the old Arab shower attendant in the bathhouse. I had been swimming at one of Alexandria's great beaches. It was the early 1970s and I was conducting tours of Egypt from California. I took every opportunity to leave my tour group and find a place to swim. I had grown used to Arab eccentricities and I stood there dripping-wet as the old man clumsily toweled over my back. Suddenly his huge hand clamped itself right down on my crotch. "Americans beeg," he repeated as he smiled toothlessly. Surprised at what he was feeling, he looked down and pulled at my foreskin. "Ah, sir! You are then a Christian?" I had learned from Burton's writings that no Egyptian youth survives his puberty without being circumcised into manhood. Experience had also taught me that uncircumcised adult men were considered to be precircumcised boys. Traditionally, uncircumcised men were considered "unclean" and were to be avoided. But, like their boys (who were encouraged to masturbate), uncircumcised men were also for play. They were meant to be masturbated.

In my job as a tour director, it was unwise to say *no* to Arab hospitality. I stood there while the old man amused himself by masturbating me. His grip was firm and he brought me to a quick, wrenching orgasm — at which point I discovered that we had an audience of five tribal bedouins who had been doing manual labor outside. They stared at my uncircumcised penis. My masturbator then became friendly and explained that he had several sons whom he masturbated to insure that their "manroots" would become large and to loosen their foreskins, thus easing their ap-

25

proaching circumcision. Then, surprising me yet again, he offered me one of his wives.

One night in Aswan my Nubian friend, Boatman Mary, invited my tour group to a Nubian dance. He met us with his *faluca* (Nile sailboat) at the steps of our hotel and took us to a sand island on the Nile. Twenty young Nubian boys from the nearby village were waiting there to dance for us. The canopy of stars in the night sky sparkled above the moonless African sky. The boys skillfully danced around a giant bonfire, singing guttural Arabic sounds I had never before heard. One small lad held us spellbound with his magnificent soprano voice. At midnight, when the entertainment ended, Boatman Mary sailed us back to our hotel and I collected money from my group for the boys.

Boatman Mary met me with his *faluca* early the next morning and we sailed to the Nubian village, so I could present the money to the town's elders. I was ushered into the place of the elders. Several old men, surrounded by boys who had followed us from the boat, greeted me warmly. They were all talking at once. I handed over the money and then asked, "Which boy had the beautiful voice?" They all yelled, "Me, me!" I described the lad to an elder. A group of boys quickly left the hut, and soon returned with the boy. I congratulated the youngster, who smiled broadly. Then to my shock, he raised his *gelaba* (Arab robe) to display his penis.

I knew that such a display was the custom among some tribes, but I didn't know how to react. I did, however, notice that he was uncircumcised. Sensing a great research opportunity, I asked about the tribe's circumcision rites: at what age were boys circumcised? Again a group of boys fled the hut and soon returned, in great excitement, displaying a small stone disc that they handed to an elder. At the sight of the disc I noticed that all the men began tugging at themselves.

The elder held the disc up for my inspection. It was a round stone gadget with a small hole in the middle. I saw faint inscriptions on it, but it was so filthy they were nearly obliterated. It was, the old man explained, the tribe's one and only such tool and evidently it had been used on every penis in the village for many generations. It hadn't been cleaned for centuries. The elder tried to describe how the foreskin tip was pulled through the small hole and then sliced off. "Not much of a circumcision," I thought, "with only the tip cut off." As I questioned the elder further, he apparently thought I didn't understand how it worked. He suddenly put the tool down in front of my crotch and said, "You try!"

I shook my head and backed away. Then there was a sudden rush of young men pulling up their *gelabas* and offering their penises for a demonstration of how it worked. To my surprise, all the exposed penises were erect. The elders, who were now yanking on their own penises under their robes, also had barely concealable erections by this time. For the first time I witnessed the group eroticism of circumcision — something Burton wrote about often. These tribal men had no reason to hide their arousal. I had read that mutually handling genitals was considered a social honor among some bedouin tribes, but these were Nubians; I didn't know what customs applied. Before I departed, they invited me to the soprano's circumcision two years hence. Such an invitation was an honor and I thanked them.

Upon our return trip on the *faluca*, Boatman Mary proudly displayed his penis to show me the result of his rendezvous with the disc. As I had expected, his circumcision seemed incomplete by the standards of my Hollywood youth. Enough foreskin remained to flap over his glans and there wasn't a trace of a scar. His glans was as smooth and moist as that of any uncircumcised man.

"With such minimal results," I asked myself, "why do they bother circumcising?" It seemed like a waste of time and, with that filthy tool, a health risk. Was it because of their religion? The Nubians in Egypt were Moslems, but that wouldn't explain the erections. I concluded that, to them, circumcision was primarily a sexual act. As it introduced them into manhood, it was probably their greatest sexual experience. At what other time in his life would the whole village concentrate on a man's penis? I hoped to return to the village two years hence. My research was rolling along.

The exotic East about which Sir Richard Burton had written with such flourish was becoming my personal land of adventure, as well. Burton was considered the Erotic Traveler and I wanted to follow in his footsteps. Why not? I was young and single, and I didn't mind being playful. I was a tour director and the natives saw me as an important link to wealthy tourists. My Egyptian cohorts felt they should be intimate with me. They saw it as good business, while for me, it was an opportunity to learn their culture firsthand. Since I was uncircumcised (and thus unclean, in their view), their "intimacy" toward me usually consisted of masturbation ... which I enjoyed. Best of all, I found that my research didn't have to be a secret here. In Egypt, unlike in America, circumcision was openly discussed.

I had one problem following Burton as "the Erotic Traveler," however: my foreskin. Burton had himself circumcised as part of his disguise when he entered Mecca. It was a daring escapade — infidels could be executed for entering the forbidden city, and an unclipped foreskin would have revealed Burton's ploy. In his book *Death Rides a Camel*, biographer Allen Edwardes quotes Burton dictating directions to the circumciser so that his penis could pass inspection by the Arabs. Thus, the Erotic Traveler spent the remainder of his life sporting an "Arab Cut" between his legs. I came to fancy myself the Erotic Traveler ... uncircumcised-style.

NOTES

1. Quoted from Richard Burton, *The Erotic Traveler* (New York: G.P. Putnam's Sons, 1966), pp. 156–158.

2. Ibid., pp. 158–159.

3. Ibid., p. 160.

3. Moslems and Christians

*B*eirut, 1973. A new tour took me to Lebanon for the first time. It was love at first sight. What beaches! Huge swimming pools had been carved out of stone on top of cliffs overlooking the Mediterranean. Swimming was the national sport; I felt like I was at home. At our hotel, the fabulous Phoenicia, my tour group relaxed in the cocktail lounge under the glass-bottomed swimming pool, watching the chorus of underwater divers perform overhead.

Beirut, with its unique blend of French and Arabic culture, was beautiful and sophisticated, both in its architecture and its people. I enjoyed sight-seeing with the tourists. But always the Erotic Traveler, I ventured down into the lobby one night after everyone was in bed. As I sipped a drink on the veranda, enjoying the lights of the harbor, I heard a low, husky guttural voice ask, "Do you like Arab men?" It was Osmonde.

Walking through the grand, palm-lined hotel lobby that night, I had noticed numerous beautiful people loitering. They were prostitutes, both men and women. Unsophisticated Egypt had spoiled me; I was used to free sex, especially as a tour guide. I decided that these gorgeous, tourist-wise Lebanese were not for me.

So I tried to ignore the handsome Arab as he repeated his question, "Do you like Arab men?" I nursed my drink, hoping he would go away. "I am wearing cologne from Paris tonight," Osmonde persisted in a deep, husky voice. "I am very good, and some people pay me much money!" He described his personal charms and listed his services and their costs. He knew he was strikingly handsome and couldn't believe that anyone would turn him down at any price. I finally explained that I was a mere tour guide and couldn't afford him. "You have rich ladies in your group?" he excitedly asked. Suddenly, our relationship became one of old-time partners. We were in business together, and he wanted me to introduce him to the women in my tour group. "We are brothers, no?"

"Some of my best friends are Christians," Osmonde repeated so often that I didn't want to hear it again. Having realized I was uncircumcised, he was determined to convince me that he had Christian friends. I couldn't have cared less. I liked him. Osmonde was just another male prostitute in prewar Beirut, but he was beguiling, sophisticated, charming ... and a scoundrel. "Do you have a rich lady friend who wants the most handsome escort in Lebanon to take her to the casino? Do you have a rich man who has never known the love of an Arab?" As far as I know, he never made a "hit" with a member of my tour group. Still, we often had coffee together. One night Osmonde eagerly offered to show me the real Beirut.

The "real" Beirut turned out to be a bathhouse. Bathhouses in that part of the world weren't remotely similar to those in America. The patrons ignored each other. They came only for hashish and aphrodisiacs. Osmonde led me into a stuffy, unpleasant room that reeked with scents. Through the haze of hashish I could barely make out forty sweaty bodies. Now what, Osmonde? I wasn't into hashish but I might sample an aphrodisiac. Expressing my preference to my friend, we moved to another part of this private hell where we came upon a group of men masturbating with great abandon. "Euphorbium," Osmonde whispered. "It cost many dollars American but it is the favored herb for the root."

When I asked Osmonde where I could get euphorbium, he pointed me to the attendant in the front office. "How much, euphorbium?" I asked the attendant.

"You are British?" the old man asked.

"No, American."

"Then your root is that of a Muslim?" he asked, looking at the thick towel wrapped around my waist. I had read in Richard Burton's books that something called "euphorbia" was dangerous for uncircumcised men, but I felt adventurous. The old man lifted my towel, gasped, and said, "Oh, monsieur, you must not use the herb. It causes the root to grow too big and makes the Christian skin sick. I, myself, have taken our Christian patrons to doctors because their little skin has strangled behind the cherry and turned black. I can offer you 'pepper.' We have 'pepper' for Christians. Twenty dollars American, please!"

I decided to ask Osmonde about this pepper stuff before I plunked down my money. Then, walking back through the bathhouse I stopped in my tracks at the sight of a European man lying back naked from exhaustion. Sure enough, he was uncircumcised ... but had been beating his penis as violently as the circumcised guys. I introduced myself as an American tour director. He said he was French, and now lived in Beirut. He was hooked on "pepper," which he pushed inside his urethra, and his penis was a swollen mess. "I plan to be circumcised and step up to euphorbium," he told me.

Tourist-wise Osmonde never mentioned my foreskin. Unlike many Arabs, he'd seen such things before. After all, he had "many Christian friends." I wanted to ask at what age he was circumcised, but he was too fun-loving a character to indulge in such serious conversation. As I packed to leave Lebanon, he asked, "You send me gifts from America?"

"Of course," I answered. "What would you like?"

"Naked magazines," he grinned.

"Okay, which magazine would you prefer? Men or women?" I laughed.

"Both," was his parting word as I got a kiss on each cheek.

✦ ✦ ✦

My next tour group was a group of aging mystics. They had planned this trip to Egypt so they could communicate with the ancient Egyptians, and they were determined to spend a night in the King's Chamber of the Great Pyramid. After placing money in the right palms, I was able to arrange an overnight stay. The Arab guards at the pyramid stared in awe as the group of forty weirdly dressed Americans entered the structure, carrying an assortment of crystal balls, tarot cards, and runestones. They climbed to the King's Chamber, rushed over to the sarcophagus, and piled their mystic toys inside the ancient burial box. Then they unrolled their sleeping bags and meditated. The small stone room was airless and damp. Fortunately, my job was to stay downstairs with the guards to be sure they didn't allow a "grave robber" to enter while my charges were communicating.

Guarding the entrance to the pyramid was a charming young bedouin with a wide smile and sparkling eyes. We spent the entire night sitting by the entrance. As the evening grew darker and the moon cast faint shadows on the desert, we could barely see groups of men strolling around on the Giza Plain. I wondered why they weren't home with their families.

Instead of answering, my smiling guard asked the buzz words, "American's beeg?" My penis was soon out of my pants and we were both erect. His penis hardly looked circumcised. A remnant of foreskin covered two-thirds of his smooth and obviously sensitive glans. He could practically cover his cockhead with skin even while his penis was erect. I asked at what age he was circumcised and I got a barrage of barely understandable information about his tribe's puberty rites ... while he masturbated.

Pumping his penis with one hand, the guard waved over a group of men with his other arm. I started to shove my penis into my pants but he grabbed my arm and said, "No!" The three young bedouins, once they took in the situation, promptly pulled out their own penises. With my guard as interpreter, I got the full story of their tribe's circumcision rites. More interesting, I was able to inspect the results and found that these fellows, all from a single tribe, had identical circumcisions. They had less skin than my guard.

Those three left, and more men were waved over to the pyramid entrance, where I again performed my inspection. Soon I could identify the tribe to which a man belonged by the length of his foreskin remnant. I had hit the jackpot. While my tourists communicated with the past upstairs, I was communicating with the present. I inspected at least two dozen modern-day Egyptian circumcisions.

✦ ✦ ✦

In 1974, after a tour with a particularly argumentive group of tourists, I was ready for a vacation and a good swim. I returned to Lebanon. On the way to the Phoenicia Hotel, my taxi driver kept going on about how we Americans had to save Lebanon's Christians. I couldn't understand much of what he was saying, but I could tell he was upset.

After checking into the Phoenicia, I began searching for my friend Osmonde. A female prostitute knew of him and said, "Oh, he was kidnapped right here. Agents from his family dragged him away. They took him back to his village to marry the bride his family had chosen." Poor Osmonde! I wagered he would slither his way out of that situation sooner or later.

With the afternoon free, I strolled along the harbor front. I was watching fishermen work their nets when a young fellow turned and walked toward me. He could have been a Mediterranean beach urchin anywhere — Italy, France, Greece — with the black curly hair, deep blue eyes, and sturdy build so common among southern Europeans. As I continued my stroll up the street, he followed me. I let him catch up and he began speaking in Arabic.

"No English?" I asked.

"No Arabic?" he replied. Able to communicate only with difficulty, I learned that his name was Amin and that he was inviting himself to my hotel room. He was a pleasant young kid and if prostitution was the only way to meet the people of this city, then so be it.

Once in the hotel he asked if he could take a shower. I thought it was a good idea. When he stepped out of the shower, I saw him naked for the first time. Foreskin! This Arab kid had foreskin!

Amin blushed when he realized I was staring at his penis. He said, "Oh, I am not ... how you say? ... slashed down there." I took off my towel to show him that I, too, was not slashed. He flashed a broad smile and, still wet, hugged me tightly. That was the beginning of a wonderful relationship.

Amin explained that he was a Christian Maronite of Turkish and Phoenician ancestry. He was a fisherman, not a prostitute. To me, he was a sudden breath of fresh air. Through all the years and all my travels, I had never been so close to another uncircumcised male. We spent the next few weeks together, touring the Lebanon he loved so much. He was proud of his country. He also proved to be a good swimmer and we hit all the best beaches. I loved Lebanon.

As we traveled around Beirut, we passed Palestinian refugee camps whose inhabitants shook fists at us, yelling in Arabic. Amin wouldn't tell me what they said, but I knew he was upset. One day as we walked to our favorite beach, passing the American Embassy in Beirut, we noticed the auto traffic had come to a stop. We finally came to an intersection where the Christian police had set up a road-block. They were searching all the cars, probably for weapons. Suddenly, they pulled four youths out of a car and threw them into a covered army truck. "Moslems," Amin said. A few days later huge guns were installed on busy sidewalks, including one in front of the embassy. For the first time in my life I felt the oppressive air of violence.

I spent my time away from Amin digging through the outdoor bookstalls near the American University. I was trying to find English translations of Arabic literature about their practice of circumcision. One day, the police asked to see my student papers. When I told them I was a tourist, they warned me to leave the country. An excited young man came up after the police left and told me that America would have to save the Christians. I invited him to coffee at a nearby cafe, where he reported that a group of Christian students there in Beirut had just been kidnapped and forcibly circumcised in a mechanic's garage. I asked, "Who would do such a thing and why?"

"The Moslems did it because they hate us and they know we are very proud of our noncircumcision. It is what separates us from them." A few days later a group of Moslem men were reportedly treated at the American University hospital because their ears had been sliced off in retaliation. The Lebanese civil war was beginning.

Amin cried as I packed my bags. I asked if he wanted to come to America. He looked at me as if I were crazy. Why would he ever want to leave Lebanon? It was, after all, his world.

In the weeks after I arrived back home in California, the news was full of the battle of Beirut. The Phoenicia Hotel had become a battlefield where Moslem and Christian militiamen fought hand-to-hand battles. Photographs depicted the bodies of Christian soldiers being pulled out of the hotel. I heard reports of surrendering Christians being circumcised, then shot, as the victors held up their hands in victory with freshly severed foreskins ringing each finger. The Moslems soon overran Amin's neighborhood, and I lost touch with him.

4. In the Shadow of the Pyramids

*B*y 1975 I had grown tired of life as a tour guide. It took too much time away from my circumcision research. I also wanted to find Amin, and I felt Cairo was the best place from which to conduct a search. I took a summer job at the Cairo travel agency through which I had been conducting my tours.

Fadlallah, owner of the agency, met me at Cairo airport. Fadlallah was a wealthy bedouin with whom I previously had been intimate. His mother was the head of his matriarchal tribe; he was her eldest son. He lived in a large, dusty home within view of the pyramids. I was put in a room with a canopied Western-style bed, installed especially for his European guests. His family slept on the floor with wooden head rockers.

The tiny, cramped travel office was stuffed with five perspiring male employees. Fadlallah's younger brother, Akabar, was the manager. Two cousins, Mohammed and Abdul, and two Lebanese refugees rounded out the staff. Khalid, a giant man with extremely wide hips, served as our outside man.

Khalid was over seven feet tall and had to weigh about three hundred pounds. He was the first eunuch I had ever known. He was the most pleasant member of the staff, and it didn't matter to anyone that he was castrated. He would have been a freak back in Hollywood, but here in Cairo he was just another respected businessman. In fact, no one even bothered to tell me he was a eunuch when we were introduced. I figured it out myself when I noticed two other equally tall men towering over the crowd on a busy Cairo sidewalk. After I pointed them out to Fadlallah, he said, "Oh, they're just eunuchs. Eunuchs are tall and wide." He shrugged. "We stopped making eunuchs after King Farouk fled Egypt. Our eunuchs are not being replaced from the younger generation."

Ladkhe, one of the refugees in the office, kept a radio blasting all day, desperately listening for news from Beirut. His family was in the middle of the battle. News and rumors about the civil war were the talk of Cairo, and refugees were pouring into the city. No one could believe that a city as beautiful and sophisticated as Beirut could degenerate into a killing field so fast. Mayhem ruled there, and I could find no trace of Amin.

Actually, I wasn't sure I wanted to know his fate, after the horror stories I heard from the refugees. One night after a festive dinner at our boss's home, Ladkhe and I were alone in the garden. Usually he was nervous and unapproachable, but this night he wanted to be friendly. It turned out he wanted me to help him immigrate to America.

Ladkhe had been working his way through college with a job at one of Beirut's many travel agencies. One day Christian militiamen burst into his office and ordered all male employees to the wall. They forced the men to display their penises. Ladkhe was the only one circumcised, thus giving him away as a Moslem. The soldiers pulled him out of the office and into an army truck. They pulled down his pants and beat his testicles with a iron pipe, finally dumping him into the gutter. Ladkhe began to cry, saying that he might never become a father. I promised to help him come to America.

◆ ◆ ◆

The fellows in the travel office were amazingly promiscuous with one another. I figured it was just a matter of male camaraderie in that part of the world. After all, the Purdah (the Moslem separation of the genders) made it difficult to have female friends ... except in the wealthier classes. Anyway, the guys kidded me about being uncircumcised and made joking gestures with knives. I laughed and took it as amusement. I learned to joke back, pretending to pull out my dick when one of them had a knife. My long-submerged circumcision fantasies were boiling to the fore. One day Abdul and I were alone and he pulled out a pocketknife and pointed it toward my crotch. I laughed, but he was serious. He pushed himself so close to me I could feel his genitals pressing up against my side, and he shoved the knife against my fly. Just then Fadlallah walked into the office and gave Abdul hell ... in Arabic. I laughed it off, but I didn't really think it was very funny.

Later, younger brother Akabar invited me to his mansion for dinner. He was a bachelor, in his early twenties, but lived in a spacious palace with male servants. After dinner, as we sipped tea in a cavernous reception room, he abruptly ordered a servant to undress me. He was my boss's brother, so I stood up while my Western clothes were removed. I felt better when he offered me the gift of a beautiful *gelaba*. Figuring the reason for being stripped was to try on the robe for size, I put my hands up so the servant could place it over my head. Instead, I felt two hands clasp my penis. The servant masturbated me while Akabar watched, smoking his water pipe. Oh well, I figured, Fadlallah must have known what his brother was doing ... he always knew everything *I* was doing.

"I wanted to see it while you had it," Akabar said as the servant dressed me afterward.

"That's an unsettling statement," I laughed, but he didn't understand my humor. He kissed my cheeks and sent me on my way. I laughed to myself as I walked through the wealthy suburb to Fadlallah's house. I was a long way from Hollywood.

While all the fellows in the office teased me about my foreskin, Fadlallah never mentioned my uncircumcised penis. I assumed it was an asset in our relationship. Homosexual relationships between two circumcised tribesmen were taboo, but uncircumcised boys and men were somehow different. I was certain that Fadlallah would have no interest in me had I been circumcised.

He knew of my interest in the subject, however, and occasionally tried to explain Moslem rites. He was very proud of being a Moslem. Together we visited the university in the ancient Khan Kahili Bazaar, where young candidates to sheikdom spend long days reciting from the Koran. I felt very privileged as we wound our way through the hundreds of chanting students. Tourists and guests were seldom allowed to enter the university's mosque and wander among these devout young men.

At lunch one day at the Athletic Club, Fadlallah ran into his friend Dr. Husseim. "Dr. Husseim will tell you everything about circumcision, my dear brother," Fadlallah crooned into my ear. The doctor invited me to his home in Alexandria.

Fadlallah allowed me to travel alone to Alexandria. He took me to the train station and waved as the train pulled out. Alone at last! Well, alone on a train crowded with tribesmen and donkeys and veiled women carrying baskets of pigeons. I was free, at least, from Fadlallah and the office crowd. I was excited about spending a weekend discussing circumcision with an Egyptian physician. I had been neglecting my research and this was my opportunity to get the real data.

In a tiny station our train pulled up next to an Egyptian military train and stopped. Both trains sat there for hours. Soldiers poured onto the platform from their train. They played around like any bunch of kids. A young soldier was pulled out of a train window and he dropped into a crowd of fellow soldiers. Soon parts of his army uniform started flying through the air. More soldiers crowded around, amid much whooping and hollering. It continued for at least an hour.

Curious to find out just what they were doing to the poor man, I rose to go onto the platform when the conductor stopped me. "Oh no, sir!" he shouted, pointing me back to my chair. When my train finally pulled out, the crowd of soldiers didn't even notice, so intently were they watching their victim. Asking the doctor after my arrival in Alexander, he said, "Oh, it was nothing more than giving the young recruit's root a rub of herb."

"You mean euphorbium?" I asked, feeling very informed about such matters.

"Of course," Dr. Husseim shrugged.

We settled down at his home with gin and tonics. He was a secular Moslem, with no qualms about alcohol. I felt good about him and was ready to ask questions about circumcision. Instead, we talked about everything else. He wanted to know all about America. His wife, who spoke only French and no English, served us a dinner with course after course and I lost count of how many bottles of wine we downed. Finally I was ready for bed.

The next day Dr. Husseim gave me the grand tour of Alexandria; we even visited Sadat's Summer Palace. My host obviously was someone important ... but he avoided discussing circumcision. I decided to relax and enjoy his hospitality. Saturday was for sight-seeing, Sunday for sleeping. I remained in my canopied bed waiting like a good guest for someone in the household to wake up. The wife finally brought me tea in bed and the doctor followed her into my room. He sat beside my bed as I sipped the tea and he proceeded to pull down my pajamas. Without saying a word, he picked up my limp penis and measured it. I couldn't believe it. Then he retracted my foreskin and took additional measurements. "Uh-huh," he murmured as he recorded the measurements. "We will attend a polo match this afternoon, Mr. Berkeley. I am sure you will enjoy seeing our best horses." He turned and left the room ... carrying with him my measurements. "Buddy boy, you are really getting a taste of the mysterious East," I laughed to myself.

◆ ◆ ◆

Amin seemed lost to the Lebanese civil war. I traced members of his family to Cyprus, where they were refugees. But Amin's name didn't appear on the Red Cross refugee list. Since the tourist season was over, I made plans to return to California, and was even toying with the idea of organizing a brotherhood for uncircumcised men once I returned home. Fadlallah invited everyone in the office to a farewell gathering in the desert. His servants pitched his magnificent tent and prepared a feast of shish kabob. As the evening began, a water pipe was passed around. We were all feeling very mellow indeed. I began to wish I wasn't leaving my good comrades. They pleaded with me not to leave, saying that I was their "brother."

The evening wore on and Fadlallah hadn't yet arrived. When I asked about him Akabar advised that he was at the train station to meet a friend. Our feast was waiting for his arrival. The guys again teased me about being uncircumcised, which I took as mere good-natured titillation. Being familiar with this bunch, I decided to do some of my own teasing. I pulled out my cock and said, "Here it is, guys, make me your True Brother."

Khalid surprised me by approaching from behind and grabbing my penis. He held me tightly with his powerful arms as the cousins pulled off my *gelaba*. I wasn't embarrassed because all these fellows knew what I had swinging, but having a eunuch playing with my cock was indeed a strange sensation. He pinned my arms behind my back and began pumping on my penis as if it were his own. I had no idea whether he had a penis of his own; I assumed he did not. The idea that someone without a penis was using mine for his pleasure was surprisingly erotic. The fellows whooped and hollered as I was pumped by Khalid's giant fist. "Wait until Fadlallah arrives, brother, and we'll see that you become our True Brother," they taunted. I wasn't sure how long I could "wait."

Akabar approached and, while Khalid held my penis still, he tried to anoint my bared glans with a white, milky glob. "Euphorbium?" I yelled. "No! Don't put that stuff on me. Please. Get your hands off my dick!" I struggled to free myself from Khalid's grip, but to no avail. I jumped as he smeared the cold, wet euphorbium into my glans. "Now brother," Akabar said, "you will not expire before Fadlallah arrives." The bastard. I felt betrayed. I also felt a wonderful sensation spread from my balls up my spine and into my cock. My organ was stretching itself out so far I thought it would burst. Suddenly, my entire being flooded inside my engorged penis and I felt the eunuch's long fingers wrapped around my soul. "My God," I wondered, "what in hell did these guys do to me? Where is Fadlallah?"

It seemed like hours passed before Fadlallah burst into the tent. He took one look at my grossly enlarged penis being beaten by the eunuch and shouted in anger, "Why have you done this to my dear brother? You were supposed to wait until I arrived with Dr. Husseim." Dr. Husseim? Did I hear right? I was struggling to compose myself when Fadlallah came over to me and said, "Brother, I have planned a special surprise for you tonight. I have invited Dr. Husseim to circumcise your root. It is my farewell gift to you." I managed a protest and Fadlallah looked at me sadly. I couldn't disappoint my best friend and benefactor. As my poor penis was relentlessly pumped and desperately needing relief, I said, "Oh, okay, circumcise me." Just then Dr. Husseim entered the tent with his bag of tools and my measurements. "Well, this is it!" I thought to myself. "There goes the foreskin club back home in America."

Khalid was still pumping me, and I wanted the sensation to last forever, especially as this was to be followed by my circumcision. The fellows, however, were getting bored and the doctor was growing restless. Suddenly, blood spurted out of my penis. Khalid let out a gasp and dropped it. The doctor inspected me and found that my frenulum had split open. He grabbed his circumcision tools and left the tent, with Fadlallah on his heels demanding his money back. Khalid followed them and I was left with a larger-than-life erection on a sore, bleeding penis, my balls aching for relief.

Only Ladkhe, the Lebanese boy whose testicles had been ruined, stayed with me. He took me to his tiny Cairo apartment. "I am sad for what they did to you tonight," he said, "it was very cruel." My sore penis was still half-erect with anticipation. The bleeding had stopped, but I was afraid to masturbate because it might reopen the wound. Realizing that I was desperate for relief, Ladkhe started to fellate me. He was less inclined toward homosexuality than anyone else in the office, and was simply helping me find relief. He was my true brother.

A few days later, I flew back to California. The only associate in Egypt I ever contacted again was Ladkhe, whom I promised to help come to America. I got him accepted into a local college, then began working on his student visa and promised to give him a room at my home. He returned to Beirut to get money from his folks ... and I never heard from him again.

5. The Uncircumcised Society of America

*H*ome again in California, I was ready to come out of the closet with my foreskin. I had seen aspects of circumcision far beyond the comprehension of most Americans. I wanted to write about my experiences and about my thoughts. However, I needed to know more. I had talked to doctors, read Sir Richard Burton, and inspected Arab penises. I had studied all the medical articles I could find. Now I wanted to know: What did American men think about the subject? Were they as traumatized by it as I had once been? In 1975 I placed several "author wants info" classified ads in underground newspapers. The response swamped me.

By early 1976, so many correspondents were pouring out their hearts to me that I couldn't handle the volume. I heard from many men who had been circumcised at birth, and resented it. "You mean that those school brats who teased me might have wished they were uncircumcised like me?" I thought. "Now they tell me!"

I was also surprised by how many uncircumcised men wrote. There *were* others like me left in America! Many admitted that, like myself, they had wondered for years whether they should get circumcised. Some who did undergo adult circumcision liked the result; others hated it. Most of my uncut correspondents believed they were fortunate to have remained uncircumcised. They wrote about the erotic pleasures of the foreskin. Not knowing what to do with all this incoming material, I traveled around the country visiting my correspondents.

One was a retired military officer who had served in the Medical Corps in World War II. His wife was an ex–Army nurse. He was circumcised at age five, and something went wrong. His urethra had been sliced open; to his lifelong embarrassment, he had to sit down when he urinated.

He was now an active anti-circumcisionist. He had already hated circumcisers when he went into the military, and he soon realized the power military medics had over uncircumcised personnel. He decided to fight. "About half of the American military personnel were uncircumcised when the war started," he told me during our two-day conversation. "The foreskins came off quickly. Most military medics of that era believed they could better control VD if they removed the foreskins of the troops. I saw many a young recruit sob as his foreskin was chopped off.

"Some officers used the threat of circumcision as a disciplinary tool. One officer in the Pacific theater had several jars of pickled foreskins that he pushed into the face of young uncircumcised soldiers, threatening to add another trophy to his collection. Uncircumcised men were often the brunt of unkind comment and ridicule as they were ordered to scat back in front of their buddies during short-arm inspections. Such regular inspections were necessary to detect VD, but dirty cocks (smegma) and tight foreskins (phimosis) often led to time on the circumcision bench. Many men just couldn't take the jokes and chose instead to give up their clean, loose, healthy foreskins. It made me sick!"

This shouldn't have surprised me, given my experience at the boys' school and later with that puny ROTC major at college. But I had no idea that a generation of men were circumcised by the military during the war. "Oh, Coach!" I thought, recalling my college swim coach, "what have they done to 'guys like us'? What's happened to our brotherhood?" My military friend insisted that I should become an anti-circumcision activist like him, using my writing skill to start a newsletter. I asked him, "Are there really enough people interested?"

"Hell, yes," he retorted. "Most of the men in America, and many of their wives, will listen up." I became an activist.

On July 4, 1976, I established the Uncircumcised Society of America as a correspondence club for men to share their ideas about circumcision ... both pro and con. I founded the *Uncut America Newsletter*, publishing the experience and opinions of club members. I published the *Foreskin Finder List*, a membership directory for interested USA members. The uncircumcised had become united.

The first edition of *Foreskin* was published in 1983 and the club flourished. In 1984 a wide-eyed, blue-eyed, blond, and very handsome student from the University of Oklahoma, after reading the book, headed for California and became my secretary. Although now an anti-circumcision activist, he was circumcised during his teens — twice. His love-hate fascination with circumcision reminded me of the need many USA members had for a "foreskins anonymous" club and he helped me start Acorn.

✦ ✦ ✦

"Tell me then," asked my circumcised French visitor, "are you now happy to have retained the foreskin you hated as a boy?"

"Well," I pondered my answer. "Yes, I am happy. For one thing, I still have the big decision before me. I still have a choice. Moreover, I'm finding many pleasurable uses for the uncircumcised penis — such as accommodating a nice Parisian penis needing the feel of foreskin."

"*Oh, monsieur, merci!*"

PART 2

A LONG HISTORY OF THE AMERICAN FORESKIN

*F*ascination with the penis has a long tradition. From the endless generations of young teenage boys who have gazed in awe at their expanding virility, to the ancient worshippers who danced around huge phallic monuments to fertility, to the curious glances stolen during army short-arm inspections or in the country club showers, the fascination has endured. Even the noun *fascination* derives from phallicism. The Romans used the Greek word *phallos* (penis) together with the Latin verb *fascinare* (to enchant) to name the *Fascinus*, a penis-shaped amulet worn as a good-luck charm. From that comes the English word *fascination*.

Phallicism has survived to modern times in many obscure ways, often as revered symbols and social practices. The valentine, for instance, originated as a symbol not for the heart, but for the testicles. At one time, Arab men laid their hands on testicles to swear the truth; that gave us the English verb "to testify."

From the phallicism of the ancient past comes the circumcised penis. The Ancients worshipped the procreative powers of the penis, which promised the continuation of life. The phallic amulet, assuring fertility to its wearer, always portrayed an erect penis (foreskin retracted) as proof of its virility. Priests, the subjects of adoration or fornication in the temples, were often circumcised to more aptly resemble the idolized erect phallus. Young candidates to the priesthood of ancient Egypt were circumcised as part of their initiation. In more "natural" societies, among the world's primitives, the circumcision rite survived as an initiation into manhood.

In today's more complex and perhaps less "natural" societies, the circumcision rite has survived for more "rational" reasons: religious tradition, moral code, social fashion, and medical dogma. Through the ages, the penis has been the focus of endless discussion and voluminous literature, theological debate and medical dispute.

The penis remains as fascinating as ever.

The enchantment of the penis has unveiled still another human propensity: man's inhumanity to man. The penis has at times become a trophy of war. The Medinet-Habou temple in Egypt, dating back to the Twentieth Dynasty, under Ramses III, depicts many scenes of the defeated Libyans whose uncircumcised phalluses are depicted in huge piles, cut off at the root. The foreskin, obviously vulnerable and possibly expendable, replaced the entire penis as a trophy by the time of Saul (I Samuel, 18:27), who requested that David bring him the foreskins of one hundred Philistines in order to gain the hand of his daughter in marriage. David, in his enthusiasm, slew two hundred Philistines and presented their foreskins to Saul "in full tale."

In more recent history, Islam introduced the custom of circumcision over half the earth, including the English-speaking nations. Today, new proselytizers of circumcision have replaced "the Sword of Islam" and in America they have had their greatest success.

The ancient phallic origins of circumcision have been separated from the modern circumcision routine. I believe it is time for us to reflect whether circumcision might be the result of our fascination with the penis, and in light of that, to reopen the debate on this centuries-old custom.

1. The British Empire Meets the Sword of Islam

More than two centuries ago, young Warren Hastings was forcibly circumcised. Along with three hundred of his fellow British workers in Cossimbazar, India, 24-year-old Warren was stripped, sodomized, masturbated, and publicly circumcised by Mogul troops who overran the British outpost. Warren watched in horror as his prepuce was carried away in a bag containing all three hundred freshly severed foreskins — trophies for the Moslem Moguls. Lanky, effeminately handsome Hastings, destined to become one of Britain's great colonial statesmen, wrote of his ordeal: "I, myself, was carved."

The incident was not the first time an English foreskin had been plucked off by Islamic warriors, nor would it be the last. In May 1751, a Colonel Law wrote in his journal, "An Englishman, Mr. Maskelyne, has fallen into the hands of Chandá Sáhib's men and I am told was vilely abused by them and forcibly circumcised. Poor devil!"[1] Ensign Maskelyne, an adjunct to Captain Robert Clive in India, was set free to walk back to his post, naked except for a bandage tied around his freshly Islamized penis. His angry superior, Clive, remarked that "even Pill-cocks [uncircumcised men] can not save their Bacon in this devillish country!"[2]

As a show of good faith, Elihu Yale, patron of Yale College and an early British trader, allowed the Grand Moguls to circumcise him. His special envoy to the Mogul court at Delhi, Thomas Pitt, was circumcised in his early twenties, as were all of Yale's young emissaries upon arrival from Britain. Effective diplomacy and bargaining required circumcised penises.

Sir Josiah Child sent two of his already circumcised men, Abraham Navarro and George Weldon, as negotiators in 1686. Weldon's journal reports,

> We were received with our hands tied by a sash in front of us when the Great Mogul escorted us into a private chamber where he ordered a Eunuch to disrobe us. He proceeded to satisfy himself we were both circumcised and therefore fitting spokesmen for an uncircumcised race. He ordered our hands be untied [and thereafter] treated us as honorable men.[3]

The Mogul rulers had harsher plans for the uncircumcised. Tippoo Sultaun, the Tiger of Mysore, used an herbal compound known as Ma'ajoon to stupefy prisoners found to have a foreskin. The aphrodisiac brought the captured penises to rigid erections. This made circumcision easier, but caused remnants of foreskin to remain on the freshly carved cocks, rendering them only partially circumcised. In the eyes of the Tiger, the incomplete clipping was a punishment as it produced only quasi-Mohammedans.

Sir David Baird, a prominent Scottish officer, met this fate along with his men. Baird and his fellow captives were seized by slaves, stripped naked, and staked to the ground, their limbs splayed wide. An old man carefully pried his long, craggy fingers into each British penis, determining the length of the doomed foreskin. Then the victim's mouth was forced open, introducing Ma'ajoon. The old circumciser patiently waited.

As the drug took effect, each officer experienced a masochistic stimulation: his teeth ground, his fists clenched, and his eyes were transfixed as he watched his penis rise in anticipation. When each soldier lay helpless and fully engorged, the old man announced, "Praise be to God! Thou art now to receive the ordinance of El-Knutneh." Slowly working his way down the line he grabbed each penis at the root. Holding it steady while its hypnotized owner watched in utter fascination, he flashed his razor once, then held the foreskin high for all to see. He then committed the severed flesh to flame as an offering to Allah.

Although circumcision is not mentioned in the Koran, the Prophet Mohammed himself is quoted as calling it "an ordinance in men and honorable in women." Some Islamic theologians have insisted that Mohammed was born circumcised. Most Moslem youths, however, waited for the ritual until they reached puberty or beyond. Arab boys often looked forward to their impending circumcision, their rite of passage into manhood, with eager eroticism. They mutually masturbated and retracted their foreskins to show each other how they would look after they became "men." Many tribes merely awaited the unscheduled appearance of a professional circumciser before they turned their boys into men. These circumcisers wandered the desert carrying a long pole skewered with dozens of foreskins ... proof of their experience.

✦ ✦ ✦

In the exotic cities of the East, colorful processions paraded through narrow, dusty streets before the circumcision of a wealthy man's son. Riding on a magnificent Arab stallion and wearing a heavily bejeweled robe, the boy was flanked by several powerful footmen who refreshed him along his route with perfumed handkerchiefs. Closely following was a stately Nubian woman upon whose head rested a copper brazier containing burning charcoal, resin, and salt — ingredients destined for the boy's penis. A group of less impressive horses followed, carrying a dozen more boys, the sons of poor men who also would be circumcised, thanks to the generosity of the rich boy's father. Singers followed, while tambourines and drums attracted a motley crowd of the curious, zealots, and those hoping for a place at the lavish reception that would follow.

The crowds, as they heard the procession approach, were never sure whether it was a circumcision or a wedding being announced. In fact, it didn't matter because the two were the same. Women to be married and boys to be circumcised were both "brides."

The two rites, circumcision and marriage, have a long connection in Moslem history. *Khitan,* the Arabic word for circumcision, is related to a group of words using the root

KH-T-N which refer to marriage: *Khatan* (father-in-law), *Khu-tana* (son-in-law), *Khutuna* (marrying). The word for uncircumcised males, *Alkhan*, derives from words referring to brides. These words appear in the same cognate forms in other Semitic languages, indicating a common ancestry in the earliest primitive Semitic tongues and (to quote *The Encyclopedia of Islam*) "that circumcision was practiced on the Arabian desert long before Mohammed was born."

In Cairo, the parallel between circumcision and weddings was even stronger. Boys facing circumcision were dressed as girls, and the parade was complete with a full entourage of wedding attendants.

◆ ◆ ◆

Historians usually theorize that ritual circumcision among Semites derived from ancient Egypt. Little is known about the daily life of the ancient Egyptians and we have no proof that they practiced circumcision. Egyptologist Alfred V. Hodenschwingh writes:

> Astonishingly, there are only seven texts in all of Egyptian literature which relate to circumcision. Although it is not clear why, the practice is almost always referred to in these ancient texts obliquely, if at all, and if it weren't for the corroborating evidence from Greek and Hebrew historians and travelers in ancient times, we might even doubt that the Egyptians practiced it at all.[4]

The Egyptian Book of the Dead, one of the seven ancient texts to which Hodenschwingh refers, refers to "the blood that ran from the phallus of Ra, after he managed to cut himself unaided." From this passage came the legend that the Egyptian God, Ra, circumcised himself, and the blood running from his penis created the world. In another of the seven ancient texts referred to by Hodenschwingh, the narrator writes: "When I was circumcised, together with 120 other men..." The most revealing of the texts, attributed to King Piakhi of Ethiopia, is translated by Hodenschwingh, "As to the king and chiefs of the lower valley, assembled to contemplate the grace of his Majesty ... they did not enter into the palace because they were impure..." Hodenschwingh explains that "this text was interpreted to mean that the men referred to were not circumcised. The word

54

'impure' is also accompanied in this text by the now familiar sign for the phallus. It thus bears witness to the strong feelings the Egyptians had about the uncircumcised penis."

If the ancient Egyptians did feel contempt for the uncircumcised penis, that is most evident in the Medinte-Habou temple of the Twentieth Dynasty. It depicts the enumeration, in the presence of the Pharaoh, of the enemies fallen in battle, including a count of the hands and penises cut off their bodies. Again quoting Hodenschwingh:

> The amputated penises piled up in this scene are those of all the enemies of the Libyan race, all those in possession of "a phallus with a prepuce." This is confirmed by the picture in which the penises ... are seen to be intact [uncircumcised]. But the hands piled up nearby come from the cadavers of the adversaries, whose penises can be seen to be circumcised. These two different procedures, officially committed as they are to the walls of the temple, show the importance that the Egyptians attached to the rite of circumcision. They were reluctant to cut off the [penis] of a man who had submitted to circumcision ... while they did not hesitate in the least to cut off the generative organs of the uncircumcised.

Whether the Egyptians were circumcised cannot usually be determined by inspecting preserved mummies, as their genitals were wrapped separately or against one of the thighs. Often the genital organs were removed from the cadaver; the penis was then embalmed separately and put inside a wood statue of Osiris. These mummified penises, however, were a favorite prey of grave robbers and are largely lost to history.

In the few mummies whose genitals did survive, Hodenschwingh reports, "The adult males were circumcised. The children were found to retain their prepuce until at least early puberty." The oldest, and most evidential, scenes of Egyptian boys being circumcised was found in the tomb of Ankh-ma-Hor at Saqqarah (Old Empire). It consists of two scenes depicting a circumcision and its procedure. The text translates: "Hold him firmly so that he doesn't move!" The figure holding the boy is shown to respond, "Begin at any time you want."

Egyptologists disagree about just which Egyptians were circumcised. According to Hodenschwingh,

> To ascertain who among the Egyptians had to submit to [circumcision] it turns out that we only have evidence from post-Pharaonic times. The specialists who have studied the documents have come to opposite conclusions. Some tell us it was a religious rite reserved for priests, i.e., that it was a caste privilege. Others declare it was originally a general and obligatory custom which at some later time fell into at least partial disuse, and that in late epochs only the priest class observed it scrupulously.

Egyptian "Coccacision"
Sketches by Hodenschwingh

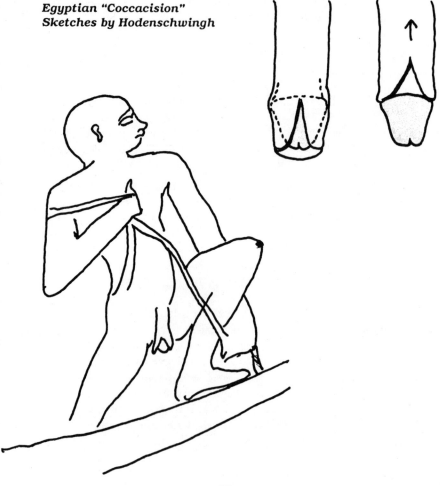

If only the finest virgin boys were chosen for the priesthood, they certainly ended up with history's most distinctive penises. A rare nude statue in Gizeh (Statue of Snefrounefer) depicts a penis with an unusually stylized circumcision. According to one Egyptologist, the Egyptian surgical rite of circumcision consisted of a simple surgical procedure: exposing the glans by slitting the top of the prepuce. The foreskin was not removed but remained intact with an inverted V, which continued partway up the penile shaft. The result was a widening of the foreskin flap with a partial exposure of the glans. Hodenschwingh named this procedure a *coccacision* (from Latin *cocca*, meaning *notch*) rather than circumcision.

✦ ✦ ✦

Egypt was not the only ancient civilization to practice sacred circumcision. According to Godfrey Higgins, a nineteenth-century Masonic researcher, the rite was performed on initiates to secret societies in "Tamal, Chaldee, Madura and Tibet." He cites an old text which refers to a Sacred Mystery School in earliest Tibet, which started the celebration of its rites with the following herald: "When we celebrate the Mysteries, we send away those who are not initiated, and shut the doors! Thy Mysteries are about to begin. Things Holy for the saints, hence all dogs [the uncircumcised]!"[5] Even great Greek scholars gave up their foreskins to enter the Mystery Schools. Pythagoras, Herodotus, Diodorus Siculus, Strabo, and even Plato reportedly returned to their uncircumcised society sporting the circumcised penis of the Learned.

This still doesn't answer the real question: How did the ritual of circumcision enter the world in the first place? Where did it originate?

The Egyptians do not seem to have been the earliest circumcisers. One of the oldest surviving pieces of Egyptian art, dating back to the First Dynasty and now kept in the British Museum, shows a battlefield with dead soldiers lying on the ground. To once again quote Hodenschwingh,

> If we regard the pictures of the victims carefully, we see that they all have been provided with a phallus which, when represented in profile, clearly shows the exposed dorsal

surface of the glans ... These men are of course circumcised, which would lead one to suppose that the Egyptians performed the procedure even in pre-Pharaonic times. But alas — the men in this ancient picture are not Egyptians: they are foreigners [who] obviously practiced circumcision *before* the Egyptians did so. Who were they? Where did they get this procedure from?

♦ ♦ ♦

Whoever they may have been, the procedure probably derived from the earliest fertility rites. Recorded fertility rites involve extensive symbolism. Allen Edwardes, for example, writes in his *Erotica Judaica* that "among Phallic-worshipping (pre-Islamic) Arabs, the Jajj was originally a fertility rite in which nude males danced around the Ka'beh (a symbol for the womb), masturbating in chorus or united 'penum in anum'..."

But in earlier times, when sex worship was in its most primitive stages, a mere symbol wasn't good enough. Primitive humans wanted the real thing. "The 'savage' does not know anything about the ovum or the sperm; he sees only the external structures involved, and deifies them; they, too, have spirits in them, and must be worshipped, for are not these mysteriously creative powers the most marvelous of all?"[6] So it was that among the earliest primitive Ethiopians the penis itself became prized as a mystical amulet.

Remote Ethiopian villagers near the headwaters of the Blue Nile warred among each other for special spoils. They sought the penises of their captives to hang over their doors. The severed penises were amulets, assuring the household of fertility. The Ethiopians returned from their battles wearing necklaces of strung penises as proof of their victory and as a present to their women.

The problem was that a penis taken from an infertile warrior brought infertility to the unfortunate house upon which it hung. Thus, the fallen warrior was masturbated before his prize was claimed to assure his captors that he was, in fact, virile. But the women in the village didn't always believe their husband's stories, and insisted that the penis hanging on their door at least *look* fertile. It had to be circumcised. After all, the foreskin was retracted when the penis was erect and a circumcised penis looked as if it was in an eternal state of erection ... and fertility.

With time, the circumcised penis came to symbolize fertility while the uncircumcised penis represented flaccid infertility. The village men, always ready to look virile, started to be circumcised. As villages merged, more and more Ethiopians were circumcised. Finally, as a sense of brotherhood developed among the growing warrior groups, they refused to castrate other circumcised men. They were forced to search further afield for uncircumcised penises, although the captured trophies were always circumcised before being hung in doorways. The warriors searched further and further down the Nile. They first discovered an ample supply of amulets among the tall, handsome Nubians of the Sudan; finally, their search took them to Egypt. We can speculate that these mountain people introduced circumcision to the Nile Valley.

While the phallus hunters of Ethiopia might have brought circumcision to our Western civilization via prehistoric Egypt, they were not the world's only circumcisers. In distant Fiji, according to the Reverend Lorimer Fison's 1884 report in the *Journal of the Royal Anthropological Institute of Great Britain and Ireland*, phallic amulets were used for other purposes. In this case, the foreskin itself became the symbol.

Referring to the Nanga tribe of early Fiji, Fison wrote:

> When a man of note is dangerously ill, a family counsel is held, and it is agreed that a circumcision shall take place as a propitiatory measure. Notice having been given to the priests, an uncircumcised lad — the sick man's son or one of his brother's sons — is taken by his kinsman to the vale tumba, or God's House, and there presented as a *soro,* or offering of atonement, that his father may recover. On the day appointed, the boy is circumcised, and with him a number of other lads whose friends have agreed to take advantage of the occasion. Their foreskins, stuck in the cleft of a split reed, are presented to the chief priest, who, holding the reed in his hand, offers them to the ancestral gods, and prays for the sick man's recovery.

Traveling still further back into time we finally reach those whom are considered to be the oldest circumcisers on earth: the Australian aborigines. Early European adventurers and anthropologists found the circumcision practices of these Stone Age people almost unbelievable. They reported that boys were not only circumcised but had their urethral canals sliced open along the underside of the penis. These boys were first noticed as having extremely wide, flat organs. They became known as vulva boys, because other men inserted their own penises into the opening for copulation. Circumcision was being carried to the full extreme of what it had always been: a mutilation.

When did these Stone Age people of Australia start cutting off their foreskins? Was it common among all Stone Age people? A rare, revealing, ages-old tale, passed on from father to son among the aborigines, gives us a remarkable clue. "The Legend of the Yaurorka, Yantuwunta, and Easter Dieri" passed from generation to generation the story of how circumcision started:[7]

> Two youths were out hunting pelicans at *peri-gundi* (a crooked, twisting place). They crept alongside the creek and threw their boomerangs at a bird that was swimming about. One boy struck his mark, but the boomerang of the other flew wide, and as they waded into the water to secure their prey, the boomerang swept past them. The young men were determined to catch it on its flight. Thus it circumcised the boy who had thrown it, and on rising out of the water he saw to his great joy that he had now become a perfect man.
>
> Upon showing his brother what had happened to him, the other youth dove for the boomerang and also emerged circumcised. The boys exclaimed to each other, "What has happened to us, for we are no longer boys, but men?" They were happy about their good fortune. Then they thought of their father who, while they became men, remained a mere boy. They found a *tula* (flint knife) and crept up to him while he slept and circumcised him. However, the father's penis grew inflamed and he died.
>
> The brothers then set out on a journey, everywhere circumcising youths and men. Coming to *Kunanana* they found that a group had gathered to circumcise some young men by means of fire. The brothers approached quietly, then suddenly sprang forward to circumcise the surprised youths with their *tula*. The crowd gathered around the brothers to inspect the *tula* and agreed that in the future,

they would make their boys into men with a knife, instead of with fire. The brothers went forward wandering through all the land, carrying the *tula*, and were everywhere honored as the benefactors of mankind.

"Originally, perhaps, a burning stick was used in [circumcisions] before it was replaced by iron," wrote early sexologist Felix Bryk.

The charring of the prepuce by means of a red-iron is as yet known only of the Nandi [an African tribe]. The Nandi take hold of the protracted foreskin, one holds it fast, another takes the glowing iron and passes it around the foreskin till it falls off charred ... If one is acquainted with the hemostatic and disinfectant result of a burn, it will not be difficult to understand how primitive man could have come upon the use of fire in circumcision.[8]

Bryk termed circumcision by fire "Circumbustion."

✦ ✦ ✦

It would be easy to conclude that the foreskin was an endangered species in the ancient world, but it found a safe haven with the people of Ancient Greece.

Classical Greece was the heyday of the male physique; and the body most adored was that of a husky young athlete with "a thin, short lingam [penis] with a long smooth tapering foreskin and gracefully hanging testicles."[9] The Greeks saw nothing indecent about nudity at their games, and in their baths young Adonises became famous for their uncircumcised beauty.

There was but one taboo: the Greek would never allow his glans to be uncovered in public. To retract one's foreskin was to appear naked. Athletes at the first Olympic games tied strings around the tips of their foreskins to ensure against any embarrassing retraction. The practice was called *kunodesme* (muzzle) or *fibula* (clasp). At times fashion called for colorful ribbons to be wound around the entire penis, which then looked like a wrapped sausage. Artificially phimosed penises were portrayed on the Classic Greek vases which recorded the beauty of the athletes. The standard for male beauty had been set for the Western World ... and it included the foreskin.

Alexander the Great's conquest brought much of the known world under Greek influence. Several Semitic, circumcising nations fell into the Hellenistic sphere. One such nationality was, of course, the Hebrews. Circumcision in infancy (not at puberty) was, to the Jews, a sacred covenant; it was the mark that set them apart as "The Chosen."

In 168 B.C., Seleucid Emperor Antiochus IV outlawed both Judaism and circumcision. Mothers who had their infant sons ritually circumcised were to be flogged, crucified, stoned, or even thrown to a pack of wild dogs. The Jewish community split between those who wanted to remain faithful to Jewish customs, and those who sought to become more Hellenized. Joshua ben-Simon and Onias ben-Joseph, rival cousins to the high priesthood of Jerusalem, informed Antiochus of their desire to adopt a "Greek way of life." They offered to sacrifice large amounts of Temple funds in honor of the Olympian gods, and "even concealed the circumcision of their genitals so that when they were naked they might appear to be Greeks."[10]

The owner of a circumcised penis encountered great difficulty trying to travel freely in the Ptolemaic-Seleucidan Empires. Men wishing to hide their circumcisions developed the *pondus Judaeus* (Jewish weight). It was a long, funnel-shaped metal or leather tube that encased the penis and clasped the remnants of foreskin. Weights pulled the skin forward. The procedure, probably less painful than surgery, was called the "burden of the Jews." In the meantime, more and more Jewish men were growing foreskins (I Maccabees 1:15, "they pulled their prepuces.") It was a particularly traumatic period in Jewish history. Then came the Maccabean Revolt, led by the Hasmonean family, during which any Jewish man or boy found with a semblance of a foreskin was forcibly circumcised. The Hasmoneans defeated the emperor Antiochus's guards, and in 142 B.C., gained independence.

The Uncovering (pri'ah) was instituted among the Jews in about 140 B.C.; it introduced to the world the tightly trimmed clipcock that would again be popular in twentieth-century America. The new Jewish leadership wanted to ensure that never again could Jewish men attempt to reverse their circumcisions. They ordered a more tightly contoured circumcision for all Jews. The newly standardized penis had none of the loose flaps of skin found on previous generations and on Arabs. In Shabbat 19:6 we read, "This shred (of foreskin) includes flesh that covers the greater part of the corona ... and if he waxes fat (and the corona is again covered) ... or if one is circumcised without having the inner lining torn, it is as though he is not circumcised."

To obtain the desired results on the circumcised penis, the *Mohel* (Jewish ritual circumciser) was instructed to seize the inner lining of the excised foreskin still remaining over the glans and, using the thumbnail and index finger of each hand, to tear it so he could roll it back fully and completely expose the glans. No skin whatsoever was to be left touching the corona of the glans. The visual result was that of a completely skinned penis, with the skin on the penile shaft becoming particularly taught and sleek during erection. The "modern, streamlined" penis which Americans, both Jews and Gentiles, came to expect on their sons, became an institution in 140 B.C. At the same time, the Romans whole-heartedly embraced the Greek concept of male beauty, in-cluding the long tapered foreskin.

The Roman Empire soon engulfed Jerusalem. At first the Romans accepted the Jewish practice of circumcision as both interesting and amusing. Jews, as well as all subjected races, were allowed to enter Rome and prosper as respected citizens. Roman society was relatively amoral at the time, and at the baths the Greek love for the "thin, narrow" penis yielded to a Roman preference for the larger, fatter cock. The long, tapered foreskin gave way to a shorter, wider prepuce that easily retracted to show off a bared glans at the orgies.

There were still those who wanted to keep their glans covered. Celsus, a Roman surgeon, gave history's first in-structions for reversing a circumcision in about A.D. 30. He wrote,

If the glans is bare, and the man wishes to have it appear covered, this can be done — but more easily with a child than with a grown man, and more easily to remedy a naturally short foreskin than for a man who was circum-cised according to the custom of certain people. With a man artificially circumcised, the skin must be detached below the glans. This operation is not very painful; as once the skin is loosened, it can be drawn back to the pubis without any loss of blood. The loosened skin is then drawn over and beyond the glans. This done, the penis is dipped frequently in cold water and covered with a poultice. As soon as it is quite free from inflammation, the penis is to be bandaged. The skin is then drawn over the glans, but kept separate from it by the poultice. In this way the lower part of the skin grows on again, while the upper part heals without adhering.[11]

While the Romans revelled in their baths, the Jews chose to practice their religion in private. The Romans became suspicious as the Jews separated themselves from the revelry, and an anti-circumcision sentiment resulted. According to Burton, "the cosmopolitan Roman derided the *verpai ac verpi* [circumcised penises as well as circumcised persons]." Claudius Rutilius Namatianus, a poet of the fifth century A.D., styled the Jew as "an unsociable animal" and all Jewry "a shameless nation that practices circumcision."[12] Anti-Semitism had raised its head and, without regard for the myriad other circumcised races in the Roman Empire such as Phoenicians and Egyptians, the stigma of circumcision was established as an evil exclusive to the Jews.

While Romans and Jews were battling out the question of circumcision, the Romans were enjoying their foreskins — and those of their slaves. Infibulation, the practice of attaching a lock or ring to the foreskin, to prevent sexual activity, came into use. Now a powerful Roman senator who spotted a well-built gladiator could purchase him as a slave, and be certain that no one would have access to the man's genitals.

An early text, *De Medinia* by A.C. Celsus (published in Florence, 1478), describes the procedure:

First of all the prepuce is drawn forward and marks are made on either side of it in such a way that, when it is released, these marks do not return over the glans. If this is tested and it is found that the marks do not return over the glans (being on the overhang instead) then these will be the place where the fibulas will be applied. After the prepuce is marked in the right places, holes are drilled with a needle and thread (much like ear piercing) and the two loose ends being tied together and run through the holes daily until these are healed, leaving only two little orifices on either side. The thread is finally removed and the fibula or clasp is attached, which should be light in character."

In A.D. 70, Vesperian instituted a circumcision tax, known as the *fiscus Judaicus* (Jewish money). Every Jewish male in the Roman Empire was subjected to an inspection of his penis and a subsequent levy. Roman soldiers, tax collectors, and other petty officials caused great indignity to Jewish men by ridiculing their penises, and on occasion even publicly masturbating them.

Once again, "prepuce pullers" came back into existence. Jewish men tried to hide their circumcisions with weights, clasps, or surgery — this time with more difficulty. Then came the final blow: Emperor Hadrian outlawed all circumcision in A.D. 131. A bloody uprising protested this edict and Simeon bar-Cocheba, messianic leader and martyr of the insurrection, told Rome that it either must tolerate circumcision or exterminate the circumcised. In the persecutions that followed, Roman soldiers forcibly drew forward the penile skin of circumcised men. Over a million Jews died at the hands of the Romans, or starved to death in hiding. Judaism and circumcision went underground.

Official opinion about circumcision soon swung to the other extreme, however. Emperor Antoninus Pius (A.D. 138–161) abolished Hadrian's ban on Jewish circumcision. His successor, Marcus Aurelius (A.D. 161–180), chose to be circumcised. Ironically it was a circumcised barbarian, the Visigoth Aleric, who sacked Rome in A.D. 410. (That Aleric was circumcised was confirmed by the scholar R.A. Lafferty: "The Gothic nobility practiced circumcision, and the commoners did not. Many primitive peoples practiced circumcision; but not many in the north of Europe, and none others as an affair of one particular class only."[13])

In the centuries that followed, the idolization of the slender, tapered foreskin as the ultimate in male beauty was perpetuated by such renaissance artists as Michelangelo, who put a foreskin on his statue of the Jewish youth David. Even infibulation continued into the Middle Ages when, according to Celsus, "it had an effect on the voice and on the state of health." Celsus gives us no indication of how the voice was thus affected, but performing infibulation on prepubertal boys was apparently thought to slow their sexual development and preserve their soprano voices for the church choir. Like the virgin boys who were chosen for priesthood in ancient Egypt, Christian Rome chose certain virgin boys for their angelic voices. Such sexual "castration" was considered healthy in a society in which celibacy was sanctified. For that very reason, some comic actors and "cithara" players wore the fibula during these times, as a symbol of their purity. Celsus admits that, in truth, such an actor wearing a fibula may be more able to sell his sexual favors. The love of the virgin (covered, uncircumcised) penis remained a preoccupation in Romantic Europe from the days of the gladiators to the days of the troubadours. Then, the "virgin" penis of Europe started its ventures into strange, and often dangerous, new lands ... in the ancient East.

✦ ✦ ✦

High Islam (A.D. 600–1000) was a period of great culture in the Moslem world. The Moslems showed more tolerance than did the Romans. In many countries, conquered populations were not forced into conversion, nor into circumcision. However, just as Rome had taxed men with circumcised penises, Islam rulers often taxed uncircumcised men. The Arab Caliphates needed the money, and a high count of foreskins was more valuable than converts.

The Moslem rulers of Christian Syria and Sicily were among the most tolerant in history. Indeed, Omar II (A.D. 712–717) even argued against religious circumcision. Only the Moors of Spain forced their Christian countrymen to shed their foreskins.

Then came the Crusades. The burly, marauding, rapine, uncircumcised knights who swept down from the European wilderness were truly barbarian in the eyes of the Moslems. Their clumsy plunder was soon met, reluctantly, with calculated cruelty ... and Islam lost its tolerance for the uncircumcised penis. Many a handsome knight was dispatched back to his cold northern woods without the benefit of his "hood." Some chose "conversion" over death upon becoming prisoners; some willingly converted. But to the European mind, circumcision remained an unthinkable atrocity.

The situation deteriorated. Five centuries later, when British colonialism set its gaze upon Moslem-ruled India, Allen Edwardes writes that

As in Biblical days, the slashed prepuces of the Unbelievers, heaped in mounds following a great battle, were held as trophies of victory in the more illustrious days of El-Islam. In accordance with the rigid martial code of the Mogul Empire, a warrior rose in rank according to the number of foreskins ... he brought in from the field.[14]

The British foreskin, that proud copy of Greek masculine beauty, had met the Sword of Islam.

◆ ◆ ◆

"By God, had I but known I was come out here to be clipped, I'd have forsworn pork and procured me a skullcap,"[15] Robert Clive remarked after the Company doctor, Dr. John Rae, cut off his foreskin. Clive, who was later to become the British governor of India, had a tight, unretractible foreskin — a condition known as phimosis. Clive argued with the doctor to save his prepuce, but Rae told him, "all Cadets who require it are circumcised, else they must give up the Company's Service."

Dr. Rae had treated many sore penises in India. Some had resulted from foreskins being whacked off by the Sword of Islam; others had been "voluntarily" circumcised to help the Company trade with the Moguls. Health was often a factor, as well. Dr. Rae wrote, "In this unwholesome Clime, venereal Infection is rampant. Morbosity feeds off the enervating Heat & Stagnation ... Mortification of the Prepuce, even of the privy Member itself, is endemic amongst the Gentoos (Hindus), who do not circumcise."

Records suggest that the Old London Company lost many cadets to such problems. Blaming the phimosed foreskin ("'Tis surprising the amount of Corruption that collects under the Prepuce," wrote Rae) the British governor and Council of Madras ordered in 1661 that "all Cadets shall be Bodily examined ... if a cadet could not strip his Yard [pull back the foreskin to entirely uncover his glans] ... [the Company doctor shall] clip the Skin entire." For the first time in history, routine and institutionalized circumcision was introduced to the English-speaking world.

For the next three centuries, Englishmen were divided between the clipcocks (circumcised) and pillcocks (with retractable foreskins that could *peel* or *pull* back). Curiosity and competition between the two styles became part of life for the British schoolboy. Clive, himself, still angered by his circumcision, was teased by pillcock cadets. According to Dr. Rae's journal, "he did menace the offending Cadets with his Pen-knife, asking who should like to be First in the Loss of his precious Skin?" Later, Clive changed his mind about his clipped penis and declared, "I am proud of bearing the mark of an empire which we may one day rule ourselves."

As the British Empire grew in might, it sent forth increasing numbers of soldiers, adventurers, and explorers. Many returned home with clipcocks. At first, these clipcocks were in the minority and bore the brunt of schoolboy indignation. By the early nineteenth century, however, the clipcock became the fashion among the British aristocracy, military officers, and others who "proudly bore the mark" of serving the Throne. The romance of the Empire builders caught the English imagination ... and the clipcock became hero.

Sir Richard Burton had himself circumcised before he entered forbidden Mecca. Burton's companion, John Speke, was circumcised on the field of battle during the search for the source of the Nile when hostile Somalis overran the British encampment. Allen Edwardes describes the scene in *Death Rides a Camel:*

> One of them shrieked, charging at Speke ... Speke parried a sharp blow that snapped off the blade of his sword ... Speke was in a daze when one of them, pressing a long knife to his throat, lashed out 'Circumcision or death, you Christian dog!' ... He pulled Speke's foreskin and stretched it tight, then sliced it off with his razor-edge blade ... The Somali ran off triumphantly with his prepuce trophy.

Speke's service to the Empire was rewarded with a magnificent statue erected in London.

As England's clipcock population grew, many a young pillcock squire, realizing how many of his peers sported their acorn (glans) unmuzzled, chose to be circumcised to better represent his privileged class. British royalty circumcised their male heirs using the finest *Mohels* in all London to do the job. The much larger English working class, however, remained firmly uncircumcised. The independent Scots, the rebellious Irish, and the Welsh likewise had no interest in "bearing the mark." Then came Queen Victoria!

To understand what is about to happen to English penises, we must reverse our history once again. Christian theology had long been struggling with three important foreskin questions: Was it possible for an uncircumcised man to be accepted into Heaven? Did the foreskin contribute to that evil called Onanism (masturbation)? And, just where was the Holy Prepuce?

The Holy Prepuce? Yes! During the thirteenth century the abbey church of Coulombs, in the diocese of Chartres, France, claimed to possess the foreskin of Jesus. It was said that the Sacred Relic gave off a sweet perfume which, when whiffed, made sterile women fertile and helped pregnant women with easy delivery. Noblewomen journeyed great distances to make pilgrimages to the abbey. One day the monks were surprised by the arrival of King Henry V's herald and messenger. Henry was king of most of France as well as England, and his French wife, Catherine, was pregnant. He demanded the loan of the Holy Prepuce. Once in London, where the Queen took a whiff, Henry returned the Relic. Catherine had an easy childbirth.

The Holy Prepuce, not surprisingly, became much in demand. The problem was, churches all over Europe claimed to possess it. In the 1715 *Dictionary of Moreri,* four major religious establishments were listed as owning Jesus' foreskin. According to one legend, Mary carried her son's foreskin with her all her life like a precious jewel, so that when the time came, he could appear before God not only in his spiritual perfection, but also in his somatic integrity.

One version of the legend claims that before her death, the Madonna entrusted this treasure to Saint John. According to another, she left it to the holy Magdalen, who left it to the apostles, who left it to their successors. From them, the Holy Prepuce was thought to have been brought to Rome by Godefroy de Bouillone, a leader of the first Crusade. Eventually, more than a dozen abbeys claimed to possess the relic.[16]

With so many Holy Prepuces clamoring for respectability, the church fathers finally had to question the authenticity of them all. Some argued that Christ must have taken his foreskin with him. A theological debate ensued: "Has Christ a foreskin in Heaven, or has He not?" Another debate followed: "Was the foreskin necessary or not?" A consensus emerged that the prepuce was no more necessary than the hair that had been cut from Jesus' head, or his nails or umbilical cord.

It was also argued, however, that as Christ was circumcised, the uncircumcised would have the advantage of him on the Day of Judgment. This possibility went against all Christian teachings. Accordingly, the clergy decided that all those in Heaven, to be equal with Christ, must submit to this circumcision before they could achieve Salvation.

Centuries earlier, St. Paul had sought to save the prepuce. "True circumcision is a matter of the heart, spiritual and not physical," he had preached, seeking to spread Christianity among the foreskin-loving Greeks. Now, the Christian fathers of Europe reversed that. They decided that the prepuce was no more important than a strand of hair needing to be cut. But this left one more problem yet facing the Church: masturbation.

Sir Richard Burton listed "the saving rite of circumcision" as one of "the thousand external functions compensating for moral delinquencies." These delinquencies most certainly included masturbation. Among Arab and African tribes Burton had witnessed uninhibited masturbation by both men and women, and especially by precircumcised boys. Burton, we must recall, was a product of a staunchly Christian-Judaic Britain. His attitude was not much different from that of Dr. Rae, in India a century earlier, who wrote, "[My Muslim assistant] tells me that Moorish boys are addicted to violent Self-abuse till they be circumcised, whereupon they are temper'd to natural Venery: which seems a mere progression to Manhood, for a circumcised Christian will indulge his folly despite the removal of its Cause."[17]

Unlike the the Arabs, the Hebrews hated the vice of onanism. Onan, the son of Judah, deliberately interrupted coition to prevent insemination (Genesis 38:9). He spilled his seed on the ground, thus committing a sin according to early Judaic law. Onanism came to refer to any form of male sexuality which didn't end in insemination, and its most heinous form was masturbation, which was considered tantamount to murder. Pious Jews would not touch their penis, preferring to support their "aim" when urinating by pushing upward on their testicles. The Christians adopted

70

the masturbation taboo and fortified it with threats of eternal damnation.

As science and medicine developed in Europe, masturbation was suspected to cause both disease and mental disorder. In 1847 a widely distributed paper was published by Dr. Vanier du Havre, the director of a children's hospital, entitled "Moral Cause of Israelite Circumcision, an Institution Preventive of Infant Onanism, and the Principal Causes of Enervation, Rehabilitation, and Reform."

At last, the notion of Jewish circumcision as an ancient evil was lifted from the European mind. Dr. du Havre's article was subtitled "Infant Onanism Combatted by Israelite Circumcision, an Improved and Painless Operation." Experts proclaimed that circumcision would hinder a boy's masturbation, making it so much work that, as his glans grew more desensitized from exposure, he would give up the habit altogether. An anti-masturbation mania spread through nineteenth-century Europe. Those marble Greek statues were still admired, but the real-life foreskins were coming off.

France and Germany both considered universal circumcision. The military classes of both countries, like the English upper classes, had long since adopted it. But to circumcise every penis in the land seemed an impossible job. Despite the claims of Dr. du Havre, they decided not to circumcise infants for aesthetic reasons; circumcision after a penis had developed its unique contours was thought to be more desirable. The Germans never decided on an age before they gave up the whole idea. The French decided on midteens; then they, too, gave it up. Victorian England did not.

Under Queen Victoria's rule, masturbation became the number-one enemy of God, and of the Throne — while also replacing Islam as the prime enemy of the foreskin. Modern sexologist Alex Comfort describes the British "masturbation hysteria" of 1850 to 1900:

> Over this period there was truly a remarkable upsurge in what can only be termed comic-book sadism. The advocacy of these bizarre [anti-masturbation] therapies was not confined to eccentrics. By about 1880 the individual who might wish for unconscious reasons to tie, chain, or infibulate

sexually active children ... to adorn them with grotesque appliances, encase them in plaster of paris, leather or rubber, to frighten or even castrate them, could find humane and respectable medical authority for doing so in good conscience. Masturbational insanity was now real enough ... it was affecting the medical profession.[18]

Dr. Thomas S. Szasz, in his book *The Manufacture of Madness*, compares this frenzy to the witch-hunts of several centuries earlier. The masturbator replaced the witch as a social scapegoat; physicians replaced the clergy as the inquisitors. One such "inquisitor," Dr. James Hutchinson, was president of the Royal College of Surgeons. His paper "On Circumcision as Preventive of Masturbation" opened the floodgates for routine neonatal circumcision. Even English working-class penises were succumbing to the Queen's surgeons.

Routine circumcision of British boys remained rampant through the first half of the new century. By the start of World War II, according to the British Dr. Douglas Baker, 80 percent of upper-class males were circumcised as were 50 percent of the working class. For the first decade, anti-masturbation prejudice remained as the rallying point for the circumcisionists.

In the second decade of the century, the medical establishment was increasingly challenged on this point, and it sought other excuses to continue the operation. The most popular one was that circumcision helped to prevent VD. With Tommy now mired in the trenches and back alleys of France, VD replaced masturbation as the favored reason to cut off foreskins. Military doctors went to work!

A few decades later, with the Battle of Britain, the loss of empire, and the coming of socialism, the tide changed again. As national health legislation was debated, a surprisingly large portion of the mostly circumcised medical establishment argued against government payment for circumcision.

Finally, routine neonatal circumcision ended with the advent of socialized medicine in 1950. At first, the upper classes continued to pay private doctors to circumcise their privileged sons. But their days were numbered. Today, England has two generations of mostly pillcocks.

For a century, the British Empire had proudly exported circumcision along with its other products. Even after the policy changed at home, it continued elsewhere. The English-speaking nations became the only Christian peoples (except the Filipinos and the Copts of East Africa) to practice routine circumcision. The hearty Australian men were about 80 percent clipped, while 40 percent of their New Zealand neighbors were. The Canadians of Ontario, much like their American cousins, were mostly trimmed; the men of western Canada and the Maritime Provinces less so; and their French compatriots of Quebec largely resisted this Anglicization of their penises. Those of British ancestry in South Africa were mostly circumcised, setting them apart from their uncircumcised Boer countrymen. Colonial Englishmen in isolated pockets around the world continued to "bear the mark." The Americans, who emerged from many ancestries, began this century with foreskin intact. But it did not last.

NOTES

1. Allen Edwardes, *The Rape of India: A Biography of Robert Clive and a Sexual History of the Conquest of Hindustan* (New York: The Julian Press, 1966), p. 77.

2. Ibid., p. 78.

3. Ibid., p. 19, quoting the *Journal* of George Weldon, and adapted into modern English.

4. Alfred V. Hodenschwingh, "Circumcision in Ancient Egypt" (unpublished). Later passages that quote Hodenschwingh come from the same source.

5. Godfrey Higgins, *Anacalypsis: An Attempt to Draw Aside the Veil of the Saitic Isis* (London: Longman, Rees, et al., 1836), p. 724.

6. Will Durant, *The Story of Civilization*, Part 1 (New York: Simon & Schuster, 1954), p. 61.

7. This story is well known in Australia, and has been told with many variations. My telling is adapted from the interpretation of Edward Karsh, *The Membrum Virile* (San Francisco: Penury Publishing, 1969), pp. 66–67.

8. Felix Bryk, *Sex and Circumcision* (N. Hollywood, Calif.: Brandon House, 1967), pp. 248–249.

9. Allen Edwardes, *Erotica Judaica* (New York: The Julian Press, 1967), p. 109.

10. Ibid., p. 110.

11. Adapted by the author from the translation of W.G. Spencer in *Celsus De Medicina* (Cambridge: Harvard University Press, 1953), pp. 420–423.

12. Edwardes, *Erotica Judaica*, p. 134.

13. R.A. Lafferty, *The Fall of Rome* (New York: Doubleday, 1971), p. 235.

14. Allen Edwardes, *The Jewel in the Lotus: A Historical Survey of the Sexual Culture of the East* (New York: The Julian Press, 1959), p. 95.

15. Edwardes, *The Rape of India*, p. 21. Subsequent quotations regarding Clive are from the same source, pp. 17–21.

16. Bryk, *Sex and Circumcision*, pp. 23–25.

17. Edwardes, *The Rape of India*, p. 21.

18. Quoted in Thomas S. Szasz, M.D., *The Manufacture of Madness* (New York: Dell, 1970), p. 192.

2. Casualties of War

*L*ess than 10 percent of the American men who fought in the Spanish-American War of 1898 were circumcised, according to Lieutenant Charles Barney in his 1903 book, *Circumcision and Flagellation among the Filipinos.*

A decade later, that figure had risen to 15 percent.[1] Masturbation mania had crossed the Atlantic. America's standard textbook for pediatrics, *Holt's Diseases of Infancy and Childhood* (1897), recommended circumcision in boys "even if phimosis does not exist, because of the moral effect of the operation." An early newspaper advertisement from a Dr. L.A. Foley of New York advertised circumcision as a cure for "laziness, pimples, paleness, association with social inferiors and restlessness in church."

American capitalism was in its heyday. America's wealthiest families traveled to Europe on fashionable steamships and hobnobbed with aristocracy. Glamorous debutantes married British lords merely to acquire titles. America's nouveau riche sought to emulate the British upper class, and one admired attribute of that upper class was the British clipcock. In England the clipcock still signified high social standing, and the sons of America's wealthy were the first on this side of the Atlantic to display the mark.

With World War I, however, the circumcised penis lost its high social standing. Hundreds of thousands of doughboys left their hearts and their foreskins in Europe. One WWI poster (recently offered for sale in the *Manly Arts* catalog of circumcision memorabilia) showed a benevolent Uncle Sam with his arm around a soldier. "Let's Have a Chat," read the headline. The brief text advised that infection and disease could be avoided by circumcision. The danger was real; a venereal disease epidemic was raging. In the tradition of their British counterparts, American military doctors decided that foreskin was a culprit.

The *Manly Arts* catalog includes another item from the WWI era: the Circumshears. This steel device came with an owner's manual stating, "The surgeon operating in a well-functioning chamber can perform fifty adult circumcisions in one hour." The military circumcision campaign of World War I gave a tremendous boost to neonatal circumcision in America. By 1920, 25 percent of American men were circumcised.

During the Roaring Twenties, infant circumcision gained popularity with the increasingly affluent middle class, which thought it would provide an advantage for their sons. Anti-masturbation sentiment reached hysterical proportions as the circumcisers cut their way through orphanages, boys' schools, and juvenile halls. One longtime headmistress at a big-city orphanage claimed, "It all started in 1919. Every time one of my boys was sent to the county clinic for the slightest complaint, he was returned to the home circumcised."[2] Another man remembered asking the nurse "Why?" as he waited in line for his school circumcision. The nurse replied, "Because that skin makes you do naughty things."[3] Medical quacks advertised such items as "Self-Circumcision Kits" and "anti-circumcision rings." The bare look was taking hold.

Another item of the period was the Original Busker's Retaining Ring, circa 1910, which was packaged in a box illustrated with a bare-chested prizefighter — the male sex symbol for that era. The ring was to be worn directly behind the rim of the glans, holding back the foreskin. According to the *Manly Arts* catalog, many surgeons recommended use of the ring before circumcision to accustom the glans to its forthcoming permanent exposure.

Listed in the same catalog is an original tattoo parlor price list. It included the cost of tattoos by hours and number of colors, and offered three categories of circumcisions: for babies, children, and adults, ranging in price from ten to twenty-five cents. By 1930, 40 percent of American men were circumcised.

America was already in a deep depression. With the collapse of the American economy came one benefit: increased access to hospital care for the poor. Clinics offered packages of several services for one price. Preventive surgery was in; tonsils and appendices were out. Entire school groups went to clinics for their removal. Quite often, the visit included an extra snip at the penis for the boys. As one man recalls, "We were all on cots that Saturday morning when two men came down the line of boys checking our dicks. I heard them yell to each other, 'This one comes off!' and 'Look at this anteater.' By the time they came to me I had an embarrassing erection. When the fellow looked at my dick he said, 'This one is okay.' I didn't get circumcised that day. My foreskin was short and when I got the least bit hard it fell back and I looked circumcised. I guess it saved my skin!" According to Thomas Szasz in *The Manufacture of Madness*, 65 percent of American men were circumcised by 1940.

Then came Pearl Harbor. Not since the spread of Islam had the foreskin faced such decimation. The nation mobilized a giant war machine almost overnight. With the mechanization of American society came an end to the tradition of giving birth at home. Circumcision was routine for boys born in hospitals. Meanwhile, American GIs were heading into battle. Unlike their sons and younger brothers, America's soldiers were still only 50 percent circumcised ... which meant the military medics found themselves face-to-face with a great many foreskins! Penicillin was not yet known, and VD was a major concern. After a battle, the medics certainly faced more important problems than foreskins, but during idle spells, it was a different matter.

A lingering anti-masturbation sentiment undoubtedly helped the campaign along. As recently as 1940, the Navy's medical regulations ordered that candidates for the U.S. Naval Academy "be rejected by the examining surgeon for ... evidence of masturbation." General George Patton had such an anti-foreskin mania that he was quoted as commenting, during a tour of an empty hospital facility when the western front was quiet, "Fill those beds with uncircumcised men and circumcise them!"[4]

Obviously, the overworked medics couldn't cut off several hundred thousand foreskins and still attend to more serious concerns. "Redundancy" became the key word. Redundant had different meanings to different officers, but generally it referred to long, tapered foreskins. Phimosis was at the top of the "redundant" list, but any foreskin that overhung the glans was a candidate. Also targeted was any foreskin, long or short, found to be covering smegma. "Short-arm" inspections included the command, "Scat back!" and any GI who pulled back his foreskin to expose a "dirty" cockhead went off to the circumciser. A war was raging, and no one had time to argue with a GI who might have different plans for his foreskin. The *Manly Arts* collection includes an undated military announcement: "Circumcision has been re-classified from elective to voluntary/advisable." As any military veteran can attest, "voluntary/advisable" meant you did it!

"There just wasn't anything else for us to do," explained a Navy pharmacist's mate who wrote to the Uncircumcised Society of America. He had aided in hundreds of circumcisions aboard ship. According to Dr. Robert Mendelsohn,

> The U.S. Armed Forces advocated circumcision because it gave an opportunity for young surgeons to practice ... Circumcision was felt to promote discipline. I presume as a result of a young recruit's learning what the Army could do to him at the outset, he might be influenced to behave himself.[5]

In the short run, however, these forced clippings created many angry recruits. "The Navy took a great deal of pleasure away from me when I was told, 'It's circumcision or court-martial,'" wrote one vet to the Uncircumcised Society of America. "My foreskin was long and tight. The medic left the room and waited for me to work it up. He wanted to see how easily I could retract during erection. It was tight but I could do it. I enjoyed the feeling of that tight foreskin rolling over my sensitive glans. Now, it's like pumping on a piece of cold, dried leather."

Another recalled:

> My experience turned me into an avid anti-circumcisionist, especially since I learned that other methods of therapy

exist for phimosis, etc. My foreskin was fully retractable, and it completely covered the glans with about $^3/4$" overhang when flaccid. When erect it would retreat behind the corona and leave a lot of play on the shaft with no discomfort whatever. I never felt embarrassed or ashamed about having my foreskin nor did I ever receive any flak from my friends. Even after I entered the Army, an occasional good-natured joke about my foreskin was all I ever heard. At age 20 I was relocated overseas and then my troubles began. I developed tonsillitis, and the medic advised tonsillectomy. I had no objection. I woke up with a sore throat and a sore penis. The medic was standing over me admiring his butchery and said, "While you were under I noticed you hadn't been circumcised, so I gave you a freebie." I called him a son of a bitch and his reply was, "You ought to thank me. I've made a man out of you."

During the war, bored soldiers often turned their attention to penises. "A major fracas among groups of soldiers stationed at the remote Aleutian Islands base resulted in the appearance of the military police...," wrote Leon Rosenhouse in his article "A Foreskin Is Missing" for *Argosy* magazine, three decades after the war. The incident occurred after the men of the base staged a "largest penis" contest. The winner was a twenty-year-old man with a foreskin so long that no other penis, circumcised or uncircumcised, could match. An argument ensued between men who agreed with the verdict and those who claimed the foreskin didn't count. Forty men ended up in a free-for-all. The winner was "called before a board of inquiry and ordered to report to the base surgeon," Rosenhouse wrote, "who decreed circumcision was immediately necessary."

Fun and games of this sort continued as the long, difficult war dragged on. Targeting Navy foreskins became a game on some ships. A USA correspondent told me one Navy medic was rumored to "entertain" the crew on Saturday nights so he could use his harvest of foreskins as bait for his Sunday morning fishing.

"When the ship crossed the dateline we always had initiation ceremonies," wrote a Navy vet to the USA.

A few days before the crossing the pollywogs [men who had never before crossed the line] were ordered to go through a short-arm inspection. Those who were uncircumcised had to write their name and serial number on a piece of paper and put it in a barrel. As the ship approached the Line all sorts of punishments were meted out to the pollywogs, but the star attraction was the fellow whose name was pulled out of the barrel. He was circumcised by King Neptunus as the ship crossed over the Line and all 1500 shipmates watched atop deck.

Confirming such antics, an ad appeared years later in the *East Village Other* newspaper offering: "FORESKINS FOR SALE! Retired Navy doctor has collection of over 900 foreskins of sailors he circumcised while in the USN. Perfect condition, preserved in a gallon bottle. Will take highest offer."

More serious excuses for circumcising GIs also emerged during the war. A jeep driver for a general reported to the USA that as he drove through the countryside inspecting installations, the general lectured his men about maintaining their "public image." In the same speech he announced that he expected all men under his command to be circumcised, and he promised a month's extra R&R in Hawaii for any uncircumcised man who immediately stepped forward to volunteer. A more serious threat was balanitis, an inflammation of the glans common in the tropics. While alternative therapies for this debilitating disease were available back home, circumcision provided the quickest cure in the jungle.

Another justification for the procedure was that while some POWs were in Japanese captivity, bamboo splinters had been nailed through their foreskins, leading to infection. For whatever causes, folly or grim necessity, the GIs came home with mostly circumcised penises to breed the baby boomers. By 1950, 77 percent of American men were circumcised.

The Korean War, fought largely by men born in the early 1930s, brought together the country's last pool of uncircumcised men. Once again, military doctors went to work. An ex-medic from that war recalled, "It was our policy to circumcise all men who reported VD and also had a foreskin, even though penicillin had made the problem easier to handle. We circumcised them after they were cured, of course." He recalled helping one young man compose a note to his wife: "I am in the hospital with a virus. I've got a surprise for you. You see, all the doctors are Jewish and so they circumcised me."

Again, GIs were mired in a terrible war of attrition. One man recalls the bitterly cold winter at the front when many soldiers were desperate to leave the war zone. When the military offered the prospect of several days in the relative comfort of Seoul, for GIs who agreed to be circumcised, they had no trouble filling the bus.

The Korean War took a heavy toll on U.S. troops, and many became POWs. One captive's experience was published in *Vector*, a San Francisco magazine with a large gay readership:

> I was held in a village deep inside North Korea. Many of the villagers had never seen a Caucasian and I was the object of much curiosity. They began to take me to their gentlemen's club in the evenings, where I was displayed naked. I supposed my penis was longer than any they had ever seen. Visitors came from nearby villages just to look at it. One night they started snipping off small chunks of my foreskin tip and keeping them as souvenirs. As new guests arrived, more of my foreskin was snipped off. My dick was sore and swollen and I had only a third of my skin left when I killed a guard and escaped ... before they ran out of foreskin!

The war finally ended, and the fifties became the golden era for the all-American boy — a boy who was cleancut of hair, of jaw, and of penis. Dr. Spock advocated that parents have their son circumcised because "it makes him feel regular." Many ethnic minorities, missed by the original circumcision bandwagon, now started sending their little squires to school with unmuzzled acorns. Circumcision tools became big business for surgical supply companies, and new gadgets flooded the market. "Self-circumcision" kits were advertised, as were anti-circumcision rings. Advertisements promised that the rings would provide all the "benefits" of circumcision without the pain of surgery.

These rings were advertised for teenage boys to wear much as they would wear braces on their teeth. The ring fit on the shaft of the penis, and trapped the foreskin behind the corona of the glans. The theory was that the glans would permanently expand once the foreskin stopped restricting it, and the expanded glans would thus trap the foreskin behind it forever.

One farm-raised man described his experience:

> My new stepfather fit the rings on me when I was twelve years old. He told me all the boys had to wear them. They must have worked because I only wore them for about a year and I've never been able to get my foreskin up over my glans since, unless I tug at it. My older brother wasn't so lucky. He was sixteen when he got fitted and I guess it was too late. We did everything we could think of to make his cockhead get fatter, but every time he took off his rings his ole foreskin would just roll back over everything. He wore the rings right up to the time he joined the Marines. They solved his problem in Korea when they circumcised him clean off.

American men who still had prepuces became a distinct minority. They faced humiliation in public showers and the trauma of being different. Like most minority groups, uncircumcised boys developed guilt complexes which, in their case, often became erotic circumcision fantasies. Emergency wards treated countless teenagers who messed up a self-circumcision attempt. One urologist estimated that such attempts were the second most frequent cause of boys ending up in his emergency care, the first being the placement of objects inside their urethra.

Parents were warning about those "bad smells," coaches were harping about "good hygiene," lovers were demanding "Get rid of it!" The experts all agreed that circumcision stopped penile cancer, cervical cancer, premature ejaculation, and phimosis — not to mention those bad smells. Some experts added that circumcision helped prevent homosexuality, and there were still grandmothers who insisted that their little grandsons be circumcised so they wouldn't be tempted to play with themselves. Some people thought circumcision to be the law. Most thought that circumcised penises were prettier and, certainly, fathers wanted their sons to look like "a chip off the old block." Everyone agreed about everything in the fifties, it seemed ... and by 1960, 83 percent of American penises conformed.

Unheard in the deafening conformity of the fifties were the first rumblings of dissent. The all-American clipcock, far from giving everyone the same cleancut look, included a smorgasbord of partial circumcisions, overly aggressive circumcisions, scar tissue, sliced-open urethras, circumcision scars, unsightly skin flaps, and unhealed nerve endings. Circumcision became so routine and perfunctory that often it was done hastily and with no concern for aesthetics. Sometimes it was done by nurses or paramedics.

Slop jobs, plus an increasing number of malpractice suits brought on by infant mutilations and deaths attributed to circumcision, brought out a few daring anti-circumcisionists. An Air Force medical officer, Captain E. Noel Preston, wrote a widely circulated article condemning neonatal circumcision in the strongest terms. He was soundly scolded by the medical establishment. However, his sickening description of a child screaming, vomiting, and defecating while being circumcised caught the attention of many young mothers.

For the first time, psychologists studied the effects of routine circumcision on the American male; one such study was left incomplete by the death of Dr. Kinsey. Even the C.I.A. investigated the effects of circumcision: "The Central Intelligence Agency conducted experiments 16 years ago on circumcised boys to determine whether the operation left any emotional after-effects, according to secret documents released Friday by the agency."[6] Perhaps it wasn't too late for the American foreskin to make a comeback. But then the nation went to war again.

✦ ✦ ✦

Unlike previous wars, however, Vietnam did not reinforce the established order. Instead, it brought a wave of protests. It became okay to question authority. Even GIs now had human rights. Nevertheless, the few remaining GI foreskins began to disappear, and for the same old reasons.

Leon Rosenhouse, in his article "A Foreskin Is Missing," reports an incident at a U.S. hospital outpost in Da Nang. An outbreak of balanitis was spreading just when the troops were desperately needed at the front. Instead of giving them time for treatment, the base surgeon ordered circumcision. Rosenhouse writes,

> The order almost caused a riot! The promiscuous soldiers regarded pending circumcision as akin to castration ... It

took several lectures by a psychiatrist to bring the recalcitrant men around. Still, there were holdouts and they were not allowed to go on leave during the remainder of their tour. It was quite a price to pay to retain their beloved foreskin.

The late sixties saw many men go AWOL, while others openly defied the draft. One USA correspondent reported, "My best high school buddy went into the military. Several months later he appeared unexpectedly at my house. He was AWOL and wanted me to drive him to Canada. I asked why he was hiding and he told me he had been detailed for circumcision and had no other way to save his foreskin. He married a Canadian girl and now has a large family up there." A few young baby boomers were finally fighting back against the military circumcisers. They were a minority, however. By 1970, almost 90 percent of American males were circumcised.

On the nation's bicentennial, July 4, 1976, the Uncircumcised Society of America (USA) was formed as a correspondence club for uncircumcised men — men long isolated from each other. It was a support group, and a platform for self-expression. The club quickly grew to over three thousand members, surprising everyone involved who had thought themselves to be "the only person who still had his foreskin." Men poured out their hearts over a subject so personal that most had never before spoken about it. Men from all walks of life, of all sexual orientations, ages eighteen to eighty-eight, and from laborers to priests, found a platform for expression about the traumas of growing up in America uncircumcised, about their love-hate fascination with circumcision, and about their opinions toward neonatal circumcision. Many were fathers of boys and some were physicians.

"I was terribly shy about my penis," wrote a USA member.

I avoided sports because I didn't want to be seen in the showers. I was considering circumcision when I received the USA material. I read it a hundred times, no less. Suddenly a tremendous burden was lifted. I was no longer ashamed of my foreskin. I started to experiment with it and found it to be a hidden treasure of eroticism. I feel sorry for the men who can't have such pleasure. I am now proud to be uncircumcised."

Self-image for the uncircumcised American improved during the seventies. Medical journals and popular magazines carried articles that questioned the advisability of routine neonatal circumcision. Young doctors at medical conventions spoke out against circumcision. A "male rights" group picketed hospitals in California with signs reading "Circumcision Is a Psychopathic Mutilation" and "The Purpose of Circumcision Is to Break the Man's Spirit Forever." Across the nation small, grassroots anti-circumcision groups such as INTACT (in Massachusetts) mailed information to young parents. For the first time, male nudity could be found in nationally distributed magazines such as *Playgirl*, and the once-hidden penis became more familiar to Americans.

At first, uncircumcised models were photographed with their foreskins retracted. The publishers didn't want to risk offending their audience with the sight of a foreskin. Readers began to complain that hiding the foreskin was not "natural." Gradually, the foreskin came forward. The "back to nature" craze had hit America.

Still another group raised its voice in the seventies: parents and doctors involved with the growing "natural childbirth" movement. As a result of Frederick LeBoyer's widely read book *Birth without Violence*, a growing number of Americans demanded more thoughtful maternity care in hospitals. Others opted for home deliveries.

How did these people feel about neonatal circumcision? Joseph Chilton Pearce, in his book *Magical Child*, gives us the answer:

> What the infant actually learns at birth is what the process of learning is like. S/he has moved from a soft, warm, dark, quiet, and totally nourishing place into a harsh, sensory overload. S/he is physically abused, subjected to pain and insult ... Consider now the male child ... they cut off the foreskin of his penis, nearly always without anesthetic. After all, the infant — suffering excessive stress, in a state of shock, and all too often with a crippled reticular formation — seems to be a vegetable, so why not treat him as one? ... remember that [circumcision] is a recent addition to our century's atrocities committed on children.[7]

In 1971, the American Academy of Pediatrics issued a formal statement declaring circumcision to be "medically unnecessary." The academy, despite a great deal of opposition in its ranks, voted to reaffirm its anti-circumcision stance again in 1975. The American College of Obstetricians and Gynecologists issued a similar statement in 1978. By 1980, routine neonatal circumcision in America was on the decline.

NOTES

1. Estimates of circumcision rates at various times are difficult to come by. The numbers in this chapter, unless otherwise attributed, come from Ronnie Anderson's book *Circumcision Pro and Con* (Los Angeles: Guild Press, 1970).

2. This incident was described by Paul Eastman, who served in the medical corps during World War II, in an interview I conducted in the early 1970s. After he retired, Eastman (who also used the name Pablo De La Rosa) spent much of his time corresponding with men who had been circumcised during the first and second world wars.

3. Incident recounted by Paul Eastman.

4. Recounted by Paul Eastman, who was assigned under Patton. Eastman recalled that his medical corps often repeated Patton's statement as a joke.

5. Dr. Robert Mendelsohn, "Circumcision," in his small-circulation newsletter *People's Doctor,* Vol. 4, No. 12.

6. From a Reuters news dispatch published in the *New York Times,* Oct. 2, 1977.

7. Joseph Chilton Pierce, *Magical Child: Rediscovering Nature's Plan for Our Children* (New York: E.P. Dutton, 1977), p. 58–59.

3. Our Search for the "Natural"

*T*he "return to nature" movement of the seventies carried over into the eighties. *Natural* became synonymous with *healthy:* Natural food, natural lifestyles, and natural bodies. Gyms replaced singles bars. And the concept of the uncircumcised penis as natural gained wide acceptance. "What I recommended to parents about circumcision in early editions of *Baby and Child Care* is quite different from what I recommend now," wrote Dr. Benjamin Spock in *Redbook* in 1989. "We now know that [circumcision] is not the only choice, nor is it agreed that it is the most sensible choice. My own preference, if I had the good fortune to have another son, would be to leave his little penis alone."

Still, the decade started with 80 percent of American boys being circumcised at birth. Most Americans, had they thought about the subject at all, would probably have asked, "So what?" One doctor summed up many Americans' attitudes when he commented on national television, "I've never heard a circumcised man complain!"

In 1984, the Uncircumcised Society of America opened its doors to "our circumcised friends and the curious." Little did we expect the flood of inquiries from circumcised men for both information and membership. Most of these men resented their all-American clipcock and wanted to know if there was some way to reconstruct a foreskin on their penis.

Another surprise, for the uncircumcised members who had felt so excluded from American "manhood," was that these circumcised men wanted to meet them — just because they had a foreskin.

"How does it feel having skin covering your glans?" wrote a married executive from New York City.

"I have always been curious about foreskin, but have been afraid to ask. I would love to have an uncircumcised man show me how he retracts his foreskin," wrote a father of four circumcised boys. "Does it hurt to have the skin pulled back?"

"I idolized my handsome father, but resented the fact that he allowed me to be circumcised. I am sure he enjoyed his body and his foreskin. He must have known what it was like for me to be deprived of my foreskin," wrote a young cowboy from Wyoming. Circumcised Americans were speaking up! Circumcision was no longer assumed to be the "natural" state of affairs.

The growing demand for foreskin restoration became a phenomenon of the new decade. The USA compiled a list of five doctors with experience reconstructing foreskins, and sent out thousands of copies to inquirers.

Several methods of reconstruction were already in use by a small number of doctors. The best approach depended in part on the amount of skin remaining on the circumcised penis.

Where some foreskin remained, a mere stretching of the skin often sufficed. And, like the weights worn by the harried Jewish men in ancient Rome, a platinum ring was placed under the remaining skin to stretch it, then the doctor placed a snug ring over the head to hold the skin in place. In a few weeks, the skin would stretch sufficiently and the ring could be removed. The final step in the modern procedure, performed by urologists, was to cut a diamond-shaped piece from the top of the opening and then sew the edges together.

The well-trimmed penis called for the "Jack Penn" operation — the description of which is not for the faint of heart. In this procedure, the skin of the shaft was cut loose at the base of the penis with a circular incision, then was inverted over the head in what was called a "degloving." The inverted skin formed the inner lining of the new foreskin. The outer layer was spliced in from a split-thickness graft taken from a relatively hairless area of the body.

A third technique was the scrotal implant method, perfected by Donald M. Greer, Jr., M.D. This was the most popular operation among USA correspondents. Dr. Greer described the method in a medical journal:

> Four separate operations are necessary for reconstruction. In the first, a turnover flap of penile skin is made for the foreskin lining and a flap of tissue from the scrotum is placed over the tip of the penis. In the second, one side of the scrotal tissue flap is divided. In the third, remaining attachments of the scrotal tissue flap are divided. A final stage completes the reconstruction with several "touch-ups."[1]

The "Phil Donahue Show" hosted one of Dr. Greer's happy patients on a 1987 TV show, shocking a normally liberal studio audience as well as millions of American viewers. The guest described how he obtained his new foreskin (scrotal implant method) and he discussed his reason for undertaking the operation. He had blamed his neonatal circumcision on his bad self-image which, in turn, led to sexual dysfunction and divorce.

"I always had pain with my orgasms," wrote another recipient of a new foreskin, "I thought it was normal. They found damaged nerves on my penis resulting from my neonatal circumcision. I had no idea what a real orgasm was like until I had one with an uncircumcised penis. My orgasms now simply blow me away!"

A woman wrote, inquiring about restoration for her husband's penis. "He has always resented being circumcised and blamed his mother. I believe that is why he seems to hate women and is very sadistic in bed."

Surgery proved too costly for many men who wanted foreskins, and for a few it was unsuccessful. It also proved unnecessary for many, who were willing to spend time and effort stretching out a new skin for themselves. BUFF (Brotherhood United for Future Foreskins) was organized as a support group and a source of information for men who were "stretching." Many men, corresponding through BUFF, reported amazing results, even on their once-tight all-American clipcock. "I now feel like a whole man," wrote one man to the USA after using the BUFF method to successfully stretch enough penile skin over his glans to form a foreskin.

BUFF used several methods to nonsurgically loosen the remaining shaft skin to the point that it covered the glans while the penis was flaccid. According to BUFF:

> Once the skin has stretched somewhat, or if you were not cut tightly, you can use the tape ring. Stretch the skin out beyond the head and wrap a length of $1/2$" tape around it to form a ring, tightly enough to hold it in place but not so tightly as to interfere with urination or blood circulation. As a rule (if correctly performed) the urine will pass, but blood circulation will be unobstructed. If the ring is too loose, it may slip behind the head and cause constriction, especially during erection. If this happens, remove the tape at once and use a smaller ring.

Using the BUFF method, one man wrote of his newly uncircumcised penis: "My cockhead is warmer and moist and I can sense feeling in it for the first time in my 30 years."

✦ ✦ ✦

While it was historically conceded that the uncircumcised penis is more sensitive than the circumcised, many advocates claimed the desensitized penis to be better. One reason often given for circumcision is the incidence of premature ejaculation among uncircumcised men.

But even on the question of sensitivity, there is no universal agreement. Sex researchers Masters and Johnson, in their tests, found no difference in sensitivity between circumcised and uncircumcised penises. Most modern researchers agree that sensitivity is such a subjective perception that it would be difficult to measure. They also agree that premature ejaculation is primarily caused by psychological factors, not by differences in penile sensitivity.

So what was everyone complaining about? Was there anything missing from the circumcised penis, besides the "superfluous" foreskin? The men belonging to the USA certainly argued that something was missing. One man wrote, "My foreskin is the best part of my penis."

A long-shelved report from the Mayo Clinic might have given us an insight into a "natural" function of the foreskin.

"Erogenous Zones: Their Nerve Supply and Its Significance," by R.K. Winkelmann, was published by the clinic in 1959. It stated:

> Two types of erogenous zones exist in the skin: nonspecific and specific ... The nonspecific regions perceive simply an exaggerated form of tickle ... It is the specific regions where one speaks of erotic sensations originating in the skin ... the rete ridges are well formed and more of the organized nerve tissue rises higher (than in other skin-type regions).

The prepuce, said the clinic, had a strong concentration of specific regions, and was responsible for a high level of erogenous sensations. In short, the Victorian circumcisers knew what they were doing. Cutting off the foreskin diminished the potential pleasure of boys who wanted to masturbate.

The S-T-R-E-T-C-H

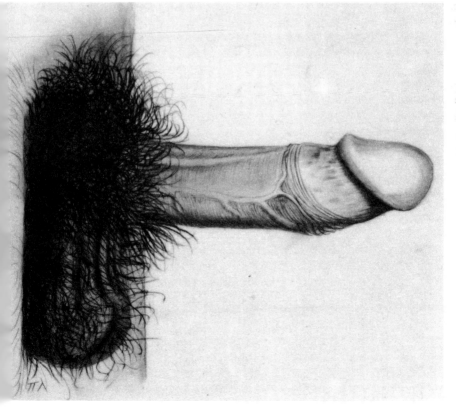

Men, during their most pleasurable moments, are not inclined to analyze the sources of their sensations, but it appears the preputial nerve endings come to life when the foreskin experiences its only possible experience; being stretched back. When that happens, the foreskin becomes a primary source of erotic sensations ... and it is loaded! Possibly, part of the impulse to plunge it in again comes from the desire for another stretch. As exquisite as the stretch sounds, much less feels, how could anyone deprive a man of such experience? All the medical, religious, and fashion excuses for circumcision suddenly become insignificant upon discovering the ultimate male experience of s-t-r-e-t-c-h.

◆ ◆ ◆

In the 1980s, the chance firing of a nurse gave the anti-circumcision movement a big boost. Marilyn Fayre Milos, R.N., was fired from her hospital job for protesting the methods used in obtaining circumcision consent signatures from young parents. The mother of three boys, all of whom were circumcised at birth, she realized that she, herself, had not been properly informed about the risks of circumcision.

With support from three other nurses, Milos started the group Informed Consent to provide better information about infant circumcision to young parents so they could make an "informed" decision for their sons. The problem of uninformed consent was illustrated by the statement of Cynthia S. Rand, Ph.D.: "Every woman who has a male child is approached and asked, 'Do you want your son circumcised?' Women just assume that, if they are asked, it must be something important and the informed-consent paper just a formality."

Milos first made headlines when she named the Prince and Princess of Wales the "Parents of the Year" in 1987 for "their decision to leave Prince William, heir to the British throne, and his younger brother, Prince Henry, intact even though their father, Prince Charles, was circumcised." Although the royal family had long been said to traditionally circumcise their heirs, at least since the days of Victoria's Prince Albert, they refused to comment on such a personal matter. It was well documented that Prince Charles was circumcised on December 15, 1948, by Dr. Jacob Snowman of London, who, according to

Charles's biographer Anthony Holden, "visited the palace to circumcise the baby."

That Charles's sons might have missed the knife was generally attributed to the determined efforts of their mother, Princess Diana, supported by her personal doctor. Her decision was rumored to cause dissent in the Royal family (the *London Mirror* reported that "the Queen's medical advisers prefer to have Princes Di's son officially circumcised by a surgeon attached to the palace.") In quest of an authoritative account of just what had happened, Milos wrote to Buckingham Palace for confirmation. She received a letter from Miss A. Beckwith-Smith, Lady-in-Waiting to H.R.H. The Princess of Wales, stating, "I regret that it is not possible to accede to your request."

Milos proved a diligent, tireless worker for the cause of stopping routine infant circumcision. She solicited and obtained the most respected medical practitioners in the nation to be on her board of advisers. She polled hospitals about their circumcision policies and questioned doctors about their attitudes. She traveled the nation, appearing on radio and television talk shows, speaking at medical conventions and at USA meetings.

Milos became the "Florence Nightingale" of foreskins, and the driving force in the anti-circumcision movement. As her fame grew, adult men poured out their stories to her in correspondence. Most of them had been circumcised and sought foreskin restoration. She published a newsletter in which, along with medical news and statistics, she chronicled malpractice suits caused by injurious or unwanted circumcisions. She was resented in the medical community because she was a woman questioning a male "manhood" rite — and "only a nurse," at that. Doctors had traditionally felt it necessary to maintain their superiority of decision over nurses. On January 1, 1986, Informed Consent became a nonprofit organization and its name was changed to the National Organization of Circumcision Information Resource Centers (NO CIRC).

NO CIRC's nonprofit status is noteworthy, because, in fact, the profit motive is often the driving force behind the circumciser's blade. The *American Medical News* announced in its January 11, 1985, edition that:

Circumcision Services, Inc., a for-profit venture launched last August, was conceived by professional marketers who have connections to the medical community. Because Houston's Harris County Hospital does not perform circumcisions on the 8,000 to 9,000 male infants born there annually, resident physicians began joking about opening a clinic for just such a purpose.

The clinic's services were marketed through a brochure included in a gift package given to new mothers.

Past generations, in contrast, were more often circumcised for medical reasons. A study conducted early in the 1900s found that Jewish women had a much smaller incidence of cervical cancer than other groups. Some researchers speculated that circumcision of the male somehow prevented the disease in women. Later studies, however, found that Amish women (whose husbands were uncircumcised) also had few cases of cervical cancer. Then the World Health Organization found an even smaller incidence of it in Scandinavian nations, where routine circumcision is not practiced.

Some doctors still argued for the knife on the grounds that penile cancer is generally unknown on circumcised penises. However, it is so rare a disease (the American Cancer Society says "no incidence rates have been calculated because of its rarity") that it hardly provided sufficient reason for circumcising millions of boys.

Today, most doctors agree that circumcision is a social rather than a medical question. A poll by NO CIRC showed that 61 percent of doctors blamed the parents for deciding to circumcise. Rather than the old reasons of health, prevention of masturbation, or prevention of "bad smells," parents cite reasons like "Circumcised penises look better," "We want the boy to look like Daddy," or "Boy might feel like an outsider if not circumcised."

A researcher confirmed this in a 1987 study. Dr. Mark Brown looked into the status of 124 boys born at St. Luke's Hospital in Denver. Ninety-nine of the babies were circumcised, and 90 percent of the boys born to circumcised fathers had the operation, compared with just 23 percent of those born to uncircumcised fathers. Brown asked about reasons for the operation, and reported that cleanliness and "not wanting their son to look different" were toward the top of the list. The only medical reason — less chance of infection or cancer — came in last.[2]

Blue Shield of Pennsylvania decided to cease payments for routine circumcision in 1987. At that time, it was the fourth Blue Shield to take such action; the Maine and Washington/Alaska Blue Shields had led the way, while California was negotiating with the medical profession. "Blue Shield has a basic philosophy of not paying for services which are not medically necessary," said spokeswoman Karen Early. "There has been anecdotal evidence on all sorts of things, but there has yet to be produced a medically sound, statistically valid study on circumcision." By 1983, the percentage of newborn circumcisions in American hospitals was down to 63 percent. It dropped to 62 percent the next year, and to 59 percent in 1985.[3]

In the meantime, with the media full of anti-circumcision news, desperate circumcised men were writing to the USA, fearing that they had been "castrated." It was not the purpose of the USA to make circumcised men feel they were missing anything. The club started because it was the uncircumcised who felt their status set them apart. It was the sad self-image of uncircumcised Americans that brought the men of the USA together; but it was the sad self-image of their circumcised counterparts that became the club's predominate concern.

Eager to help all our members improve their male libido, the USA quickly consulted several members who were urologists and formulated a reply:

> According to most modern physiologists, circumcision rarely interferes with the function and pleasure of the penis. The erogenous mucocutaneous region of the foreskin is not totally lost on most American clipcocks. The inner lining of the foreskin, the most erotically explosive skin area, is not cut entirely off in many of today's circumcision methods.

As we explained to many of our worried members, in modern circumcisions, much like in those of ancient Israel, the inner lining is stripped back over the skinned shaft and laid bare, inside out, and sewn into that position. Thus, many circumcised USA members report that the area between the glans and the circumcision scar is their most sensitive. During masturbation many circumcised men merely touch this area alone (and not the glans) to achieve an orgasm. They put pressure on those supererotic nerve endings that remain on their penis. It works. A college student wrote: "I dig the looks of an uncut cock on another man, but my sleek cut cock is not only beautiful, it gives me and my partners much pleasure, I just wish I had the choice of circumcision for myself. I probably would have chosen to be circumcised. I'll never know."

Happily, many "cut" men, writing to the USA of their resentment at being circumcised without their consent, at the same time offered the opinion that they had the greatest penis on earth. I learned from members with a physiology background that the reversed foreskin area of the circumcised penis usually retains some of its original erogenous sensitivity, even though nature meant it to remain an interior organ in a warm, moist pouch. The exact area of greatest sensitivity varies. Some circumcised men report that this is the frenulum area (on the underside of the glans); others say it's their circumcision scar (where sensitive nerve endings were opened and became scar tissue).

These small areas of intense sensation certainly provide the circumcised man with adequate erogenous feeling to enjoy his penis, but the thought that this area could have been much larger haunted many circumcised USA members. After all, many had witnessed teenage friends masturbate by rolling their foreskin with long, sweeping strokes over the entire length of their penis. "I fantasize having a long foreskin which remains forward over my glans when I am erect," wrote a college professor. "I'm sure I would experience greater sexual enjoyment if I had the sensation of skin rolling over my glans-penis. Just the thought of having a long foreskin is enough to get my poor skinless cock stiff!"

"The glans penis is wasted on most circumcised penises," a New Zealand naval medical officer wrote to the USA. There's no simple, objective way to measure glans sensitivity, but I've asked USA members to tell me their perceptions. Members with tight foreskins usually reported the most sensitive glans; they were often moist, even wet. Those with looser foreskins had drier and less sensitive glans. Circumcised men differed widely with their report of glans sensitivity; some reported glans that "would explode" if touched while others admitted, as one man wrote of his cockhead, "You can pound it with a sledge-hammer before I feel anything there."

"[Circumcision] takes away an area of skin whose underside, which faces the head of the penis, is a mucous membrane, as is the head of the penis," wrote Tim Conway in a magazine article.

> After circumcision the skin of the glans loses its mucous quality, becoming more like the skin of the rest of the body. Dr. [Thomas J.] Ritter claims that this desensitizes the head of the penis: "Even if it means only a loss of anywhere from 5 to 11 percent of the nerve endings, it is still a loss of sensitivity in one of the most sensitive areas of the body."[4]

Against this growing anti-circumcision sentiment, the foreskin faced a new health threat in the 1980s: AIDS. Persistent reports suggested that uncircumcised men stood a greater chance of contracting the dreaded new disease.

In 1986, Dr. Aaron Fink wrote to the *New England Journal of Medicine:*

> My own clinical observations, supplemented by those of other urologists, indicate that the redundant prepuce may be as long as 7.6 cm in some cases. Thus, the inner mucosal lining can represent nearly 50 percent of the surface area of the shaft when the penis is erect, thereby increasing the risk that AIDS will be acquired through a skin break.

He was commenting on a report from microbiologist William Cameron that uncircumcised men in Kenya were nearly ten times more likely to contract AIDS from heterosexual exposure than were circumcised men. Dr. Fink theorized that the foreskin's inner lining was susceptible to tears that could allow the AIDS virus to enter the bloodstream from an infected partner. Heterosexually transmitted AIDS had already reached epidemic proportions in Africa.

"It is my hypothesis that the presence of a foreskin predisposes both heterosexual men and homosexual to the acquisition of AIDS,"[5] Fink concluded in his letter. The following year, he asked the California Medical Society to pass a resolution confirming the medical necessity of "newborn circumcision as a public health measure." Dr. Fink wrote to his colleagues that "after four thousand years of anecdote, rancor, and rhetoric, I believe the time has finally come for the alleged medical benefits of a newborn circumcision to be determined by credible and critical debate among clinicians and either clearly expressed or rejected as myth."[6]

Marilyn Milos of NO CIRC rejected these arguments, and aggressively counterattacked. "Recent reports in the media on the transmission of AIDS through even slight blood contact have caused concern among parents about whether infant circumcision increases the risk of AIDS to the child, to sexual partners," she retorted.

> The concerns are threefold: Is the high AIDS rate in the U.S. and Africa linked to the high number of circumcised males in both [of those] parts of the world? About 85 percent of the world's males are uncircumcised, especially in Europe and Asia where AIDS cases are few. Does the circumcision scar and loss of protective genital tissue make abrasion and fluid transfer more likely in circumcised males? Can AIDS be transmitted through blood contact while diapering a circumcised infant during the 7 to 12 days it takes the wound to heal?

> "We contacted over 100 AIDS researchers," Milos continued, "and despite circumstantial evidence, no studies have been done on AIDS and circumcision." Meanwhile, medical experts questioned the reliability of the Kenya report. One pointed out that most men in Kenya were circumcised, except for those who had left their tribal circumstances, thus avoiding their ritual tribal circumcision, and these men mostly lived in urban poverty, where they faced an increased threat from AIDS. Nevertheless, the possibility that the foreskin increased a man's susceptibility to AIDS was serious enough to cause the American Academy of Pediatrics to reconsider its 1975 anti-circumcision decision.

◆ ◆ ◆

While medical debates whirled around foreskin, a new group raised its voice in the Uncircumcised Society of America: Men wanting to be circumcised. Many uncut Americans fantasized about being circumcised, or about other men being circumcised. Most speculated that their fantasies resulted from growing up among circumcised peers. They were masochistic about their foreskin, probably resulting from the childhood guilt about being different. But at this point in their lives, a mere trip to the urologist wouldn't be enough. They wanted to be circumcised in the context of male camaraderie. When the USA responded to these fantasies by publishing forced-circumcision fantasy fiction, other members (mostly those circumcised at birth) vehemently complained. One fantasy series involved Sarge, a military drill instructor and notorious prepucephobe whose motto was "You can't make a Marine out of a skinhead!" Resounding complaints about Sarge caused me to cancel the series.

The uncut men with a love-hate fascination of circumcision formed Acorn (from the Latin for *glans penis*), their own support group. Despite all the advice to the contrary, the urge to have an adult circumcision played a relentless role in the sexuality of these men. "I just want to know what it's like to have an all-American clipcock swinging between my legs before I die!" wrote one fifty-year-old man.

"To me, the word *circumcision* is powerful! I love the word," wrote a young husband. A lumberjack wrote us: "I do not consider myself gay. Except for the circumcision fantasies, my sex life is hetero. I have never talked to another man about circumcision, but the thought of doing so makes me so hard it hurts." And from a computer engineer came this: "I would love to watch my penis being circumcised, and getting together with a bunch of fellows to compare circumcision scars would fulfill my most erotic dreams."

Acorn received a great deal of mail from men with an erotic interest in circumcision. In its newsletter, the club announced, "We now have developed a line-up of men seeking to join our SIRcumcision festivals. If your penis tells you to join our club, please write."

One man wrote to Acorn:

I am mainly interested in supporting your club as it contributes to the eradication of that anatomical catastrophe, the foreskin. A circumcised cock is the epitome of masculinity, the triumph and crowning glory of the mature male. Dr. Willard Goodwin called the circumcised penis "a beautiful instrument of precise intent" as opposed to the uncircumcised penis hanging between the thighs in apparent shame and modesty, hiding and covering up the male's true self.

Acorn found support from a long-standing advocate of circumcision: the U.S. Army.

A ten-year study, led by Major Thomas E. Wiswell of the pediatrics department at Brooke Army Medical Center in Fort Sam Houston, Texas, gathered statistics about 427,000 infants born in U.S. Army hospitals over a ten-year period. In 1987, Wissell announced the results in *Pediatrics* magazine. According to this study, as the circumcision rate fell from 85 percent to 70 percent during that decade, the rate of urinary tract infections (UTI) rose correspondingly. Wiswell reported that "this increase was due to the overall number of uncircumcised boys, whose infection rate was 11 times greater than that of circumcised boys."[7]

Here, Wiswell claimed, was "at least one medical benefit" for circumcision. UTI was a potentially life-threatening condition in infant boys, and Wiswell's article sent the medical community into a huddle. A group of Swedish doctors wrote that "soon there may be pressure for a program of circumcision of babies in Europe where, until now, circumcision has been rare except for religious reasons and among certain of the British upper classes." The American Academy of Pediatricians came under pressure to ease its earlier opposition to neonatal circumcision.

Once again, the anti-circumcision forces mobilized in response. And once again, Marilyn Milos threw the ball back into their court. "Circumcision causes UTI," Marilyn Milos headlined in her newsletter.

> Three pediatricians in Israel report that in their study of Jewish infants with fever in the first month of life, 17 percent suffered from urinary tract infection. "UTI appeared a few days after circumcision. The high incidence of UTI following circumcision in our patients could indicate that the procedure itself causes the infection by local edema and urine retention," report Dr. J. Amir, et al., Beilenson Medical Center, Petah Tikva, Israel.

Milos was backed up by Oregon pediatrician Martin S. Altschul, who examined the records of all infants under one year of age with UTI admitted to Kaiser Hospital in the

Northwest from 1979 to 1985. He concluded that only one-tenth of one percent of uncircumcised male infants had UTI. He wrote in *Pediatrics* that this rate is "far too low to justify routine circumcision of all males.... There must be either a methodological difference or a pathological difference between my data and [Wiswell's Army report]."

The American Academy of Pediatrics also found flaws in the Army study:

> Studies in Army hospitals are retrospective in design and may have methodological flaws. For example, they do not include all boys born in any single cohort or those treated as outpatients, so the study population may have been influenced by selection bias.... In the absence of well-designed prospective studies, conclusions regarding the relationship of urinary tract infection to circumcision are tentative.

The jury was out.

On April 8, 1988, Region 9 of the California Nurses Association presented Marilyn F. Milos with its highest honor — the Maureen Ricke Award — "for her dedication and unwavering commitment to righting a wrong" and her work on behalf of children "to raise public consciousness about America's most unnecessary surgery." The First International Symposium on Circumcision took place March 1 to 3, 1989, co-sponsored by Marilyn's NO CIRC and the prestigious Institute for the Advancement of Human Behavior. The same co-sponsors presented the Second International Symposium on Circumcision in San Francisco from April 30 to May 3, 1991.

As we entered the last decade of the century, a new generation of uncircumcised young men was joining the USA, this group having little problem with their self-image. They were proud to be "uncut." The ratio of cut-to-uncut in school showers shifted. By 1990, NO CIRC estimated that 40 million Americans (35 percent of the male population) were uncircumcised. The circumcision rate in hospital births had fallen to 59 percent, with the western states reporting a mere 42 percent. In other English-speaking countries the percentages of the male population that was not circumcised ranged from 98 percent in Great Britain; 78 percent in Australia; and 75 percent in Canada. Worldwide,

85 percent of men were uncircumcised.[8] By the year 2000, "most American boys will be intact like their grandfathers," writes Milos. "Will we then wonder what all the fuss was about?"

NOTES

1. "Foreskin Reconstruction: A Preliminary Report," by Donald M. Greer, Jr., M.D., and Paul C. Mohl, M.D., in *Sexual Medicine Today*, April 1982.

2. Reported by Edward Edelson, "Just Like Dad," in the *New York Daily News*, August 10, 1987, p. 137.

3. The circumcision rates quoted here were gathered from hospitals by NO CIRC.

4. "The First Rip-Off," by Tim Conway in *Hustler* magazine, May 1979, p. 94. I know that some readers will question the use of *Hustler* as a source; however, this was a solidly researched article, sent to me by a USA member, about a subject all too rarely discussed in more mainstream magazines.

5. Aaron Fink, M.D., in a letter published in the *New England Journal of Medicine*, October 20, 1986, p. 1167.

6. Quoted from a "Dear Friend and/or Colleague" letter dated January 1987.

7. Associated Press, "Infections Trouble Boys Not Circumcised," in the *San Francisco Chronicle*, March 20, 1987.

8. All figures in this paragraph are from NO CIRC polls, as reported in the organization's newsletters.

PART 3

DEAR BUD: CIRCUMCISED AND UNCIRCUMCISED

"Dear Bud," the letter was addressed, "My lover wants me to get circumcised. I don't want to lose my foreskin, but I am in love."

"Forget it!" I answered. "If you have a problem with your penis, consult a urologist. If you have an erotic desire to get circumcised, go for it! If you are sacrificing your foreskin to satisfy another's whim, from the consensus of letters the USA has received about similar situations, I think you're in danger of not only losing your skin but also your lover. Too many times the circumcision proves to be a disappointment and the relationship breaks up ... leaving you with a skinless cock. You accepted your lover as he came packaged. Why can't he accept your original packaging? Educate him and make everyone happy."

Such letters poured into the USA mailbox. Once I had founded the Uncircumcised Society of America, I found it impossible to respond to all the correspondence I received.

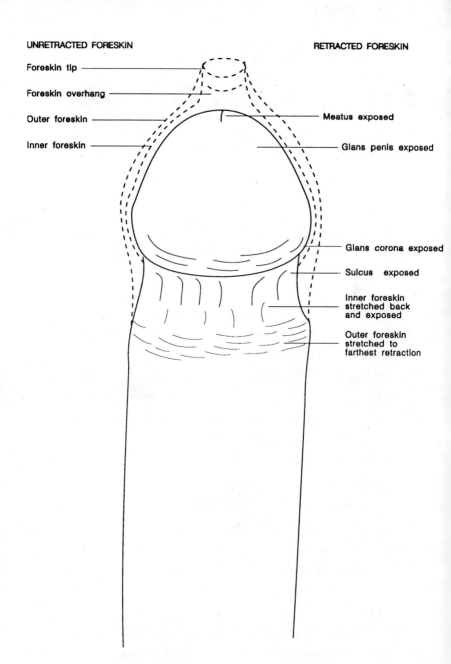

UNRETRACTED FORESKIN

Foreskin tip

Foreskin overhang

Outer foreskin

Inner foreskin

RETRACTED FORESKIN

Meatus exposed

Glans penis exposed

Glans corona exposed

Sulcus exposed

Inner foreskin
stretched back
and exposed

Outer foreskin
stretched to
farthest retraction

It was unfortunate, because many correspondents had serious questions — about their sexuality, and in particular, about their penises. To those with questions that seemed urgent, I did reply. I advised them that I was not a medical doctor and that, if they had a medical problem they must consult a urologist. I explained that I was merely a writer and investigator, researching a story. But when I could, I was happy to share my experience, as one male to another.

In my answers, I referred to the experiences that other correspondents had reported to the USA. Doctors, researchers, and clergymen were among those writing to us and I often benefitted from their advice. However, the unanswered mail continued to stack up.

Several general topics surfaced as the chief concerns of my USA correspondents: the stretching of foreskin to make it longer; foreskin restoration; phimosis and other foreskin problems; the advisability of adult circumcision;

smegma; and "where can I meet uncircumcised men?" A love-hate fascination with circumcision seemed to prevail, as well as a curiosity about foreplay with the foreskin. There was virtually no literature to be found on these subjects.

Hoping to satisfy my unanswered correspondents, I initiated a question-and-answer column. The column appeared in several USA publications and also in three nationally distributed magazines. These columns, in turn, generated additional mail, some of it from women.

In the pages that follow I've selected the most important and interesting of these questions and answers, often updating my original responses with new information. I've also added some new questions, which have never before been addressed in print. Please be warned that this section is sometimes explicit, and it often involves some homoeroticism. It has been my experience that frank questions need frank replies to be meaningful.

1. Stretching It, Smelling It, Loving It

*D*ear Bud,

There is both aesthetic and erotic attraction in the uncircumcised penis. The glans penis is a vulnerable, secret, and precious thing to be shielded from easy public view, protected from danger of abrasion or desensitizing contact with flesh or fabric, revealed only to the intimate. To see it blatant and surrounded by scar tissue is an ugly profanation.

The flaccid unmutilated penis is an object of natural beauty, graceful and elegant, framed and focused by the junction of the torso and limbs, the symbolic center of the male body. The fully engorged penis is not aesthetically so elegant and graceful but demonstrates a state of aroused desire both exciting and awesome, a necessary prelude to ecstasy and fulfillment.

The most erotically stimulating visual image is that of the moment when the glans is just at the point of projecting from its sheath, stretching against its confinement, about to emerge in a display of potency and power. As in ejaculation the sperm is involuntarily propelled through the penis from deep within the body by a galvanic combination of physical and psychological forces, so with the natural penis, in the promising precursor of orgasm, the glans is propelled from its protective shield and emerges as under the mastery of an irresistible erotic force made palpable and visible.

The circumcised penis is denied this exciting transition. Engorgement does not radically change its aspect but merely enlarges the penis and makes it rigid in a continuous process, without the mini-climacteric of emergence.

There is a vast difference in appearance between the circumcised and the uncircumcised flaccid penis. There is only a subtle difference between the circumcised and uncircumcised penis when erect. At the stage of almost full erection the change is about to take place in the natural penis, and this is, erotically, a moment of truth and wonder and delight.

Name Withheld by
Circumspection

Dear Circumspection,

Thanks for such a glowing testimonial to the beauty of the uncircumcised penis. Unfortunately, most Americans still seem to prefer the looks of the circumcised penis, judging from the persistently high neonatal circumcision rate in this country. The appearance of the penis is still touted as a good reason to cut off foreskins. As psychologist Karen Ericksen Paige notes:

> Some doctors even argue that circumcision should be done for purely aesthetic reasons: a penis without a foreskin, they say, is more pleasing to the eye, neater and less likely to produce bad odors. One physician, Willard Goodwin, wrote that "circumcision is a beautification comparable to rhinoplasty [a nose job]."

Circumspection, one might question your emphasis on the visual aspects of the penis. Who cares about the "looks" of a man's penis? After all, who's going to see it? Well, besides the importance of a man's self-image, the current health crisis has forced many people to develop new safe-sex practices in which visual perception plays a more important role than penetration.

Dear Bud,

Your literature saved my foreskin and I'll thank you for that as long as I live. I had grown up feeling insecure about my uncircumcised penis, thinking it to be a sign of immaturity — a "little boy" cock.

I never felt that I was a real man around my circumcised peers. I graduated from college last June and was engaged to be married soon thereafter. I had planned to get circumcised sometime during last spring so that my cock would be healed and ready for action on my wedding night. Well, I found your book *Foreskin* under the bed of my college roommate and read it fervently from cover to cover. When I read in the book about the erogenous nerve endings in the foreskin and how they give off sensation when the foreskin is pulled back over a rigid shaft, I had to pull my boner out and give it a test.

You were right, Bud. I realized immediately that the backward motion of my foreskin gave me the greatest erotic sensation and the forward motion over the head the second greatest sensation. Needless to say, I had to jack off and did so that night with a full appreciation for my foreskin for the first time. What an orgasm I had! I immediately canceled my circumcision appointment. I wasn't about to deny my bride the best cock I could give her. The honeymoon isn't over yet.

Hot Husband

Dear Hot Husband,

Hey, Hot, thanks for the testimonial. Your description of that foreskin *stretch* really does it justice!

Dear Bud,

As a circumcised man who has had a lifelong fascination with uncircumcised cocks (even though I am a married heterosexual), I must ask you this question: What does it feel like having foreskin on your penis?

Circumcised Man

Dear Circumcised Man,

You can't believe how many times this question is asked by USA correspondents. Well, how do I answer it? The foreskin is just there ... like your finger or your ear. You don't feel it unless you think about feeling it. However, roll the foreskin tip between your thumb and finger and you do get a tingling sensation. Pull the skin back just slightly to urinate, and you get an added, pleasant sensation to an otherwise boring bodily function. Skinning it back further, rolling it over the sensitive surface of the glans, you'll probably get an erotic sensation that makes you want to completely uncover your penis. Under the right circumstances, this total stripping of the foreskin generates enough sensation to cause the penis to stand up and take notice.

During erection, while the shaft is hard and the glans is flaring, the uncut man receives his most exquisite experience as the skin stretches out its nerves to accommodate the engorged penis. The best sensation comes as the skin slides down over the shaft. This sensation is felt in both masturbation and coition. And from their perspective, many women who have written to the USA get turned on by the sensation of the penis sliding in and out of its "glove" of foreskin. The rest of the time, however, the foreskin behaves itself ... it's just there.

•◇ ◇•

Dear Bud,

I am a nineteen-year-old college student and a virgin. I came here from a small midwestern town where all my peers were circumcised. I joined a fraternity here along with nine other pledges. We took a few showers together but I kept my eyes straight ahead because I certainly didn't want my fraternity brothers to think I was gay. Then one night at dinner a senior stood up and said, "Do you realize we have pledged the first uncircumcised fellow the house has had in five years?" They asked me to stand up and take a bow. They cheered and applauded and whistled. I nearly died!

I am not sexually aggressive and hoped to avoid sex at the fraternity house altogether. But since the dinnertime announcement I have had no less than five of my brothers ask me to pull out my dick so that they could get a close look at it. One of them, a senior, asked me to jack off for him. My roommate, who was a fellow pledge, woke me up one night by fingering my dick. He wasn't embarrassed at all. We got into a mutual jack-off. Bud, are these guys putting me on? Are they gay or are they really just curious about my foreskin?

Virgin

Dear Virgin,

Curiosity and contention between owners of the two styles of cocks goes back generations. One writer recalled the following episode from his career as a British schoolmaster:

> Twenty-one of the boys, stark naked, were lined up against their lockers, and the remaining boy was going down the line, examining his friends' penises very closely, fingering each one lightly in order to satisfy himself of the presence or absence of a foreskin. Those with foreskins he dubbed Cavaliers; those without foreskins he dubbed Roundheads ... He explained that they were organizing a game of Roundheads and Cavaliers for whiling away the afternoon.[1]

Virgin, some of your fraternity brothers might be gay, but so what? I don't really think their curiosity about your uncircumcised penis is unusual. Mutual masturbation will certainly not change your orientation one way or the other. You didn't say what your orientation is, and apparently, it makes no difference to your fraternity brothers. They sound like great guys and, obviously, they like what they see. I hope you're no longer embarrassed by being uncut, because I think you and your foreskin have found an appreciative home.

Anyway, the following passage from a letter to the USA illustrates how even hunky athletes are human. They too are curious.

> I was the only uncut player on the team. Being professionals we were always on the road and, like it or not, we saw a lot of each other's equipment. My foreskin sure got a lot of long stares in the showers. Nothing was ever said but I felt sort of odd about it and wondered what the fellows were thinking about my dick. One night in a hotel room I was awakened by a strange movement in the room. I sat up and realized it was my roommate jacking off under his covers. He was a 240-pound bruiser and the poor guy was so strong he couldn't take care of himself without shaking the room apart.
>
> Realizing I caught him in the act, he smiled and said, 'Can't stop now!' I rolled over pretending to show no interest but he was getting hotter and whispered, 'Hey man, you hot too? Feel like rooting? Hey, I've always been curious about

that dick of yours and how that skin works. Want to show me?' My dick was full-up when he turned on the light. He bent over from his bed to get a close look while I slid my foreskin up and down over the full length of my dick, covering the head and then exposing it. He almost stopped stroking himself. Suddenly, his mammoth fist tightened its grip around his fat cut tool and his stroke got fast again. He turned out the light and we both finished ourselves alone. Nothing has ever been said about that night. He's straight as hell.

●◇ ◇●

Dear Bud,

My uncut dick is beautiful. It is the long, slender, cylindrical type with long, loose foreskin which comes to a pointed tip, even when it is fully erect at about 7 $^1/_2$ inches. I always get compliments for it and one of my friends asks me to strip when I visit for an evening of TV and he just stares at it by the hour.

Recently, because of the health crisis, I have been into mutual masturbation. A real hunk gave me a call because he heard I was uncut and he'd never had an experience with foreskin. I found his circumcised cock easy to pump. After all, I've had plenty of experience with skinned dicks. But he just couldn't get the hang of it with my dick. He finally said, "Your foreskin is in the way. Why don't you get circumcised?" I was shocked. No one had ever before asked me that question. How should I have answered?

Cylindrical

Dear Cylindrical,

Your penis sounds like a classic to me. So, you want an answer to why you should keep it that way? Okay, here's a list of reasons most uncircumcised men want to hold onto their foreskin:

1. Your foreskin is loaded with all those super erogenous-producing nerve endings. Who wants to lose those?

2. Your foreskin protects the glans from abrasion and loss of moisture.

3. Foreplay. There is so much more that you and your partner can do with a long foreskin. You can prod fingertips into it, stuff toys inside. You can spread it out and share the warm, moist skin with your partner by placing your overhang over her nipple, or his cock. (The latter activity is currently the rage; it's called "docking.") After an hour or so of foreskin foreplay, love should surely be consummated most happily.

4. Penis fashion. Foreskins are in, as you have experienced. The long, pointed foreskin is the fashion for the men of the nineties. Why do you think everyone, even circumcised fellows, are stretching out their penile skin?

5. Masturbation. Okay, so your date couldn't figure out how to pump your foreskin? He can be educated. Actually, pumping on an uncircumcised penis is easier than beating most cut cocks. The long sheath of skin is nature's pumper. It provides a rhythmic, unabrasive sliding motion. The uncircumcised man usually doesn't need lubricants on his penis, either.

6. Versatility. If an uncircumcised man wants a change in his action, all he has to do is retract his foreskin. Masturbating with the foreskin held back can give new, exciting sensations. The super-sensitive glans really flares out with direct action over its moist surface. Just remember to allow your foreskin to roll back over the cockhead when you are finished, to protect the sensitive, erogenous glans.

●◇ ◇●

Dear Bud,

I enjoy your column. Several times you've mentioned foreskin retraction, which doesn't work for many uncut men. But an uncut guy can still have the normalcy and handsomeness of a bare glans, standing out there for all the world to admire, even without circumcision. I've perfected a method on my own cock. Here's how:

1. Don't pull the foreskin back. Leave it alone.
2. Just hold the foreskin gently with the thumb and index finger of one hand.
3. With the thumb and index finger of the other hand, reach

in and gradually pull the glans, and also pull the inch or so to which the glans is joined (the sulcus), out and down (in tune with the force of gravity).

If an uncut guy does this as often as possible for at least three months he'll get fabulous results, and even the bonus of a longer penis. But he must never stretch his foreskin, as it would be counterproductive. You may want to pass this information along to your readers. Why hide the steak?

Bare Head

Dear Bare Head,

Head, some of my readers would dispute your contention that a bare, naked glans looks normal and handsome. Well, maybe handsome ... but what could look more normal than a long, drooping, dangling foreskin over the tip of the penis? Of course, I understand why you use that term. When we were growing up, glans were bouncing all around the school showers and they sure looked normal. Most uncut boys, back then, longed to have a dick that proudly displayed the "steak," but as hard as we tried to push the foreskin back off the head, the damned thing would just creep back to cover up the works. It's a different story today, my friend, because long foreskin is in fashion.

Having said all that, I must confess that your method is intriguing. I've yet to meet a man who didn't enjoy playing around with his sex, and most of us are always open to a new sensation. I suppose if an uncut man can keep his foreskin shoved back off his cockhead for three months, his skin will stay retracted more easily. The glans always flares out upon orgasm, and if the foreskin doesn't roll back to its natural position, the glans often remains enlarged. I'll admit it feels great having that fat, wide steak hanging out there ... at least temporarily.

The success of retraction really depends upon the anatomy of the penis. A flared-out corona (rim of the glans) can trap the foreskin behind it. Remember the Original Busker's Retaining Ring that I described earlier in this book? It worked on the same principle. Some men are born with a wide, bulbous glans; if they escape circumcision, they often end up with either a short foreskin or one that appears permanently retracted. Other men, with a slender glans and loose, long foreskin, would have a difficult time staying retracted even after three months of tugging. There is, of course, a huge variation in penises and the relationship of the foreskin to the glans varies widely. One physiologist wrote that he considered the two parts of the penis to be independent functioning organs, each with its own purpose.

A 1960s survey of the penises of West German army recruits gives a clue to the natural distribution of foreskin types. The survey was conducted to determine which men were more likely to be found with smegma — those with tight foreskins or those with long, loose, ones. The survey categorized 3,000 men between the ages of eighteen and twenty into five foreskin types: (A) no visible foreskin, (B) short foreskin, (C) long foreskin, (D) tight foreskin, and (E) phimosed. Out of the 3,000, only 258 young Germans were group

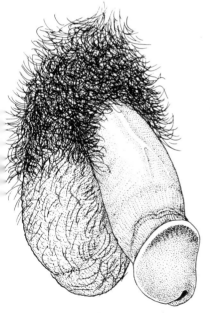

Type A: No visible foreskin

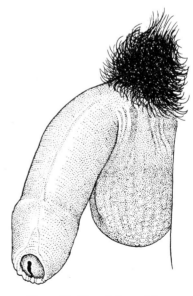

Type B: Short foreskin

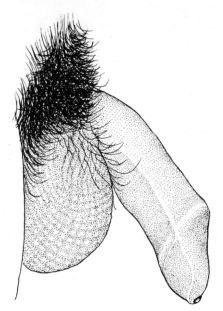

Type C: Long foreskin

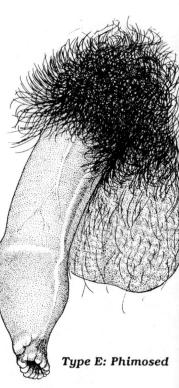

Type E: Phimosed

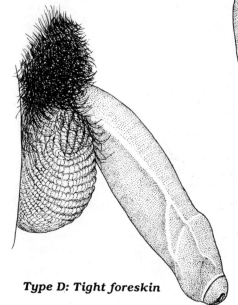

Type D: Tight foreskin

116

A and of those only a quarter had been circumcised (probably because of childhood phimosis). Half of the 258 had such short foreskins that they had long since fallen behind the corona and in the rest, it was impossible to determine whether they had been circumcised. Group B (short fore-skins) included 1,258 men (42 percent). Group C (long foreskins) had 1,236 men (41 percent). Group D (tight foreskins) had only 181 men (6 percent). Group E (phimosed) included only 82 (3 percent).

From this list, your method will probably work for group B and possibly, with a lot of work, group C. So, what the hell! Let's give it a try! It could be sort of a nostalgia trip, taking us back to the good old days when those bouncing steaks were the rage.

●◇ ◇●

Dear Bud,

I have a one-inch overhang. How can I add another inch or two? My partner digs the look of an extra-long foreskin.

Not Enough Overhang

Dear Not Enough Overhang,

Easy. The foreskin is made for stretching. After all, it must accommodate the rise and fall of the penis, and you'll find that stretching it proves enjoyable. Some skins, of course, are more easily stretched than others. With an inch of overhang I'll bet your skin is the loose, long type and already used to stretching action. Another inch or two should be a piece of cake. I can think of six possible ways to increase your overhang:

1. Cotton balls. After bathing in the morning put some lubricant on your glans and then, bringing your foreskin forward, stuff as many sterile cotton balls inside as you can fit. The lubricant will keep your glans from chafing. You'll find that you can stuff more and more cotton inside each day. If necessary you can tape your foreskin shut with surgical tape, keeping the cotton locked in. It will feel great, as if your cock is floating in air. Keep the cotton in there until the next piss.

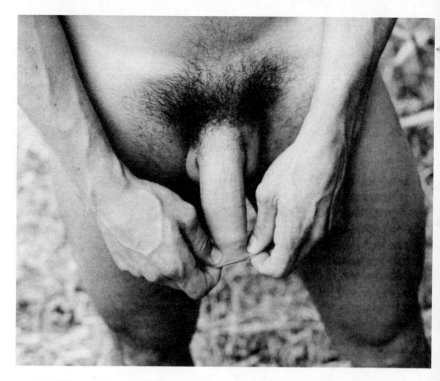

2. Manual stretching. Cut and file your thumbnails, then push your thumbs inside the foreskin and pull them apart. Gradually, you'll be able to stretch further without hurting. If you get tired of solo stretching, find a friend with good thumbs and strong biceps. Some doctors recommend this type of stretching for youths with tight foreskins.

3. The Donald Duck. The chromium gadget sold in medical supply houses as a "vaginal speculum" is exactly what many doctors use to stretch out the moderately tight foreskins of young patients, especially in England. It works! With a strong grip on the handle it will stretch out the skin perfectly. One variation is to lock it into a wide position (but not so wide that it hurts), then tape the instrument to your skin with Dermicel tape. It will act as both a weight and a stretcher. Wear it while cleaning the apartment in the nude on Saturday morning and you'll have plenty of extra skin for your date on Saturday night. Just don't catch the handle on something, unless you have self-circumcision in mind.

4. Rubber washers. Find a washer with a hole that is just the right size to pull your foreskin tip through ... and let it dangle there. It makes a comfortable and effective weight. It's also easy to pull off when you need to take a leak. Many types of gadgets can be used as weights either attached to the foreskin or ringed around the sulcus (behind the glans). You must be careful, however, not to use anything that causes irritation. If it does, remove it fast.

5. Teeth. This method usually requires the help of a second person. Grab your cock at its base and push all that skin up front until it just looks like a wad of bunched-up gum. That will give your friend plenty of skin to suck up as it stretches out along your partner's molars. Relax and let your friend chew gently ... no need to bite! Most foreskins love to be gently chewed and they'll stretch themselves out for more. Caution: While chewing foreskin is most probably "safe sex," just make sure the chewing doesn't get you too excited (it seldom brings an uncut man to orgasm) and be honest about your HIV status.

This method can be tried solo, provided other parts of the anatomy allow. The USA received this letter from a yoga instructor: "We practice celibacy at my ashram in California. What my Guru doesn't know is that celibacy is no problem for me because I have several positions which allow me to place my mouth on my cock. We wake up at 5:00 a.m. and in the privacy of my tiny room, I chew on my foreskin while I meditate. I never retract my foreskin except for cleansing and my foreskin has become my most erotic part. All I do is gently teeth it to the rhythm of my chant and I have an orgasm. No one would ever know because I keep my foreskin locked shut by clenching my teeth until I reach for a towel. I think I have discovered the secret of why so many Holy Men in India have extra-long foreskins. Mine is now 3 inches flaccid and getting longer."

6. Jacking off. Yes, masturbation is Mother Nature's way of keeping the foreskin loose, limber, and healthy. Most urologists report that tight foreskins are caused by their patients not doing their "homework."

Dear Bud,

I don't understand why an uncut guy would want to train his foreskin to stay back off his cockhead. He might as well be circumcised. Some of those guys seem to have cockheads just as dried up as cut guys. Recently I visited a gymnasium in Amsterdam and was shocked to see so many of them with retracted foreskins and dried cockheads. What gives?

I'm one of those guys who keeps his foreskin forward at all times and that is where I prefer it. I even piss with my foreskin forward. I allow the stream to go right through the funnel. It feels good that way and I have no problem with my aim. I would never be seen in public with my glans exposed, not even at a public urinal. I am not a prude and enjoy nudity in the right places, but with my glans uncovered I feel naked. With my foreskin forward I feel clothed, even if I am only in my birthday suit.

Up-Front Foreskin

Dear Up-Front Foreskin,

Yes, pal, one of the nice things about being uncircumcised is that we have a choice. We are convertible. We can either keep our tops up, down, or anywhere in between ... or, at least, make the attempt to do so. Felix Bryk theorized that uncircumcised men have a subconscious desire to retract their foreskin because it feels good. To feel the stretch of the foreskin permanently would be just wonderful, but it doesn't work that way. Still, when the foreskin is back off the head, it's reminiscent of sexual arousal. Bryk theorized that the "urge" to be circumcised is a result of the desire for that "magic moment" to last forever. Of course, there's a flaw in that logic — you can't keep enjoying that stretching sensation once the organ that provides it has been chopped off. But uncut men all over the world seem to find it erotic, or manly, to retract in public.

Up-Front, the point in your letter that really caught my eye is your feeling of nakedness when your foreskin is retracted. The ancient Greeks had the same attitude, tying strings around their foreskin to insure that their glans wouldn't pop into public view. The Eskimos, who traditionally practice nudity in family situations, tie strings around their foreskins for the same reason. A German anthropologist named Sitzflisch has even theorized that the human practice of wearing clothes derives from the foreskin covering the glans.

Writer Eichelschutz Hautlob elaborated on this idea in a recent magazine article:

> Since nothing springs from the human mind except those things already patterned by nature, the idea of clothing came from the only natural covering the human body possesses (other than eyelids, etc., which are controlled by motor reflexes), which is the foreskin, and early man perceived both the foreskin and clothing to be sexually enhancing.[2]

Hautlob claims we adopted clothing not for protection from the elements but for the purpose of "erotic intensification" — in other words, to look sexy.

His thesis is buttressed by the progression of coverings worn by those Stone Age groups still living. Some Melanesian Islanders wear only the most elemental form of clothing. They merely insert their prepuced glans (with foreskin forward) into seashells and consider themselves fully clothed. Of course, the colorful seashells merely encourage the viewer to imagine what is being hidden. The next step in clothing can be found among other Melanesians, whose clothing consists of penis-wrappers. The entire penis is covered with leaves or leather and they are fully attired, even with their scrotums fully exposed.

Next come the Papuans of New Guinea, who insert their penises into long gourds and wear them in an upright, erect position. The Indians of eastern Brazil take clothing one step further, suggesting both an erotic need for clothing and a utilitarian one. They tie their foreskin overhangs shut with beautiful bows of netted cordage; both protecting their glans from injury as they walk through the jungle and drawing attention to their penis.

Well, Up-Front, you get the picture. Paris is a long way from Melanesia but their fashions apparently come from the same pattern — the foreskin.

Dear Bud,

I am towing around a lot of scars about my dick. I grew up on a farm, so as a kid I wasn't around other children much. The only boy I knew was my younger brother. What got me off to a bad start was one hot summer night when we were sleeping naked, I happened to wake up and what did I see? My kid brother's dick was standing right up in the air in the moonlight. I couldn't believe it! It was a hell of a lot bigger than mine. I tried to imagine having such a big cock. I figured it was because he was circumcised. I decided mine was smaller because I never got circumcised.

One night our cousin came down from Savannah. Being how that bedding space was scarce, guess who ended up in my bed? Right. It was my cousin, who was just my age. I had a hell of a time sleeping while he was in my bed, and one night I was awakened by something poking my back and it was annoying the hell out of me. I put my hand behind me to see what was going on and, fuck, I grabbed on to a dick larger than I had ever imagined existed. I felt around just enough to figure it was circumcised too. I just felt terrible.

Now, here is my point, this size thing has been the biggest thing on my mind night and day. I went out to the family doctor and he said just relax and make do with what I have, even if I don't like it. He told me my dad had an uncircumcised penis like mine and I should discuss it with him. Hell, dad never let anyone ever see his dick and he wouldn't talk sex to anyone. So, I've tried penis pumps, vitamins, and some exercises I read about, but the little fucker only pushes out to a puny five and a half inches to this day.

Now, here is my question. Should I get circumcised like my brother? Would I then have a big dick like his? You see, I just turned 21 and have a hankering to go into town and get some sexual acts but I'm afraid of being laughed at because of my little dick and being uncircumcised.

Little Fucker

Dear Little Fucker,

Hey, kid, give yourself a break. You might have a smaller dick than your brother and cousin, but you have one thing over them: you still have your foreskin. Someday you'll thank your father for that. You're too young and inexperienced to appreciate your endowment from God. The right partners will not reject you and when you find the right partner, you'll forget all about "the size thing." Who cares whether your brother is larger than you? The gene pool in a family offers several sizes and shapes of penises. It also offers qualities of beauty, of character, of health, and so on. Gadgets, penis-pumping machines, and exercises can temporarily pump up a penis to its particular limits and possibly keep it there, but it's possible to injure yourself or to desensitize your penis while you experiment. I don't recommend it.

Circumcision does not make a penis larger. As one urologist wrote, "How can cutting off something add anything?" Yes, the circumcised penis does seem to have a larger cockhead, especially around the coronal ridge. Some men who experience adult circumcision report a slight expansion of the glans. Often the expansion is more imagined than actual, as the naked cockhead is synonymous to an erect penis in the mind's eye. Anyway, Little Fucker, your $5^1/_2$-inch penis is not small, it's a good, healthy average as American dicks go. Vernon Bosch, in his book *Sexual Dimensions*, states that 90 percent of all men measure between $4^1/_2$ and $7^7/_8$ inches when erect. There are a hell of a lot of circumcised dicks out there smaller than the one you're worrying about. So, think about it. Do you really want some of that five and a half inches whittled away?

I am sure that as time goes by, you'll realize that the "scars" you're towing around are in your head and will go away with maturity. At least, the scar is not on your penis, where it would never disappear.

Dear Bud,

I've heard you mention the aphrodisiac Ma'ajoon. I'm into aphrodisiacs but that is a new one to me. What is it? Do you know about euphorbia? I understand the Arabs use it. I bought a euphorbia plant and smeared the sap onto my glans but it burnt me so bad my cock peeled. Where can I get the same euphorbia plant that the Arabs use?

Feel Like a Peeled Dick

Dear Peeled Dick,

Ma'ajoon is mentioned in the notes of Sir Richard Burton's translation of *The Arabian Nights*. According to historian Allen Edwardes, it's made up of "hemp, milk, melted butter, poppy seeds, datura [a plant yielding atropine and other drugs] and sugar." Yes, *stay away* from our local species of euphorbia. Euphorbia is a huge genus of plants (which includes the poinsettia) whose milklike sap is toxic to the skin. I know firsthand what even the sap used in the Mideast can do to a penis. While the preorgasmic titillation might be incredible, the "hangover" is a sore, irritated cock.

Edwardes described roaming bands of professional marauders,

> operating from Morocco to Timbuktu to Libya and the Sudan, who take great pleasure and delight in the genitals of their victims [whom] they capture by ambush ... then they carefully inspect and analyze the captured genitals — they fondle, measure, compare and take photos. Then, they eagerly smear the irritating juice of the euphorbia plant on the captive's glans, stake the naked prisoner to the desert floor by one ankle and retire to sit in a circle to watch the resulting action.

The captives, who might be soldiers or merely unfortunate travelers, had no choice but to masturbate themselves furiously, to the joyful whooping and hollering of their tormentors. "The prisoners pound on their cocks with primitive abandonment," according to Edwardes. "If the captives happen to be uncircumcised, they are usually relieved of their foreskins which, after being stretched and violently manipulated over grossly enlarged glans, are sore and willing sacrifices to Islam."

Today in America, with our free access to erotic literature, we don't need such drugs to get us off. Besides, what can be more erotic, or safer, than watching your own handsome penis in action?

●◇ ◇●

Dear Bud,

You might think this is a letter about "a friend" and it is, in fact, about a very good friend. My friend has a phimosis (unretractable foreskin) condition and his embarrassment is so bad that he's actually ashamed of his cock. He's got seven inches hard and is a great-looking guy. He's been to doctors about it and they uniformly recommend complete circumcision, but he doesn't want to loose his skin. Who would? This fellow's foreskin absolutely will not retract; when he has a hard-on the skin is stretched tight over the glans and ends in a tight pucker. The pucker begins with a tight, fibrous band of darker tissue and ends with about $^1/_4$ inch of loose overhang. The phimosis ring is so tight that you can't even stick your index finger up past it. His piss stream makes a slight flare and his semen sort of oozes out of the pucker. This condition makes him "piss-shy" and he holds a towel in front of himself in the locker room. Some of his potential sex partners have made cruel, derogatory remarks about his condition.

Bud, have you heard of anything besides circumcision that might help my friend?

Phimosis Friend

Dear Phimosis Friend,

I certainly have. I recommend investigating the dorsal slit. This surgical procedure is used by many urologists to avoid performing a complete circumcision on a phimosed patient. It is a mere vertical cut down the topside of the foreskin. It loosens the tight skin and heals, in most cases, to an almost unrecognizable scar. However, many factors could be responsible for your friend's condition, and he should talk with a qualified urologist to determine whether the dorsal slit would help in his case. Tell him to shop around persistently to find the *right* doctor — one whose first reaction is not circumcision. In a few rare cases, circumcision is the only effective therapy for phimosis, but in most cases, the dorsal slit does the job.

While phimosis is not the most desired condition and can lead to serious health problems (including bladder infection from backed-up urine) and a stationary foreskin misses out on the *stretch*, it certainly should not be the cause of embarrassment or derogatory remarks these days. Many members of the USA (mostly circumcised members) are fascinated by phimosed penises, and consider them to be most erotic, because they're the opposite of their own skinned dicks. The USA has several phimosed members, one of whom wrote an article for a USA Newsletter describing how he cleaned out his tight foreskin with Q-tips. We were swamped with mail from readers saying that it was one of the most erotic articles they had ever read. So, Friend, tell the fellow to ignore the derogatory remarks — he's got admirers out there — but to keep looking for the right urologist.

The USA has another phimosed member, a married naval officer. His skin is also absolutely stationary. In his case, the foreskin is actually attached to his glans, and the Navy decided not to circumcise him because of the potential complications. Hell, the fellow fathered six healthy children with his immovable dick. He might not be able to experience the *stretch*, but I can imagine that the entrapped, super-sensitive glans does feel the movement of his foreskin, and he must like it. In any case, his phimosis certainly doesn't slow him down. He's got a partner in every port.

Such a condition isn't always the fault of nature. In a newborn baby, the foreskin is often still attached to the glans. The two may not separate until a boy is several years old. Parents or doctors who retract an uncircumcised infant's foreskin prematurely can cause scarring, and, later, phimosis.

Unfortunately, this happens all too often. Many parents are told that if they don't allow their baby to be circumcised they'll have to clean out his penis ... an unwanted task for some parents. Even if they take the trouble to scrub out the foreskin, what is in there? Smegma? Smegma (the substance that forms in the preputial space) doesn't appear until puberty. Most pediatricians believe that the prepuce should be left alone until after the preputial space has formed at the age of three or four years. At that point, the foreskin can be comfortably retracted over the glans, and the child should be taught to clean himself.

Dear Bud,

Mom was always after my older brother to clean out his foreskin. I idolized him, and his big full-skin dick was magical to me. But Mom hated to be bothered with cleaning his peter when he was little so I guess that's why they got me clipped when I came along.

When he was about fifteen and I was ten, we were drying after showers when Mom walked into the bathroom. She pulled his foreskin back and found smegma. She game him hell. Alone again, he said, "Shit, I can't help it. It's there no matter how many times I wash it out. Mom just doesn't understand dicks." Well, I didn't understand his dick either, and his smegma was an intriguing mystery.

One night he was out with his school buddies and had too much beer. He took off his clothes, then fell asleep on a chair. My curiosity got the best of me. I quietly sneaked over to him, pushed back his foreskin, and there it was! I was looking at smegma up close. The smell of it almost made me high. It was my brother's smell. I quickly went to my room, got a leather pouch, returned to my brother, and scooped out his smegma.

My best-kept secret, from both Mom and my brother, was that I kept the smegma in the pouch and enjoyed a whiff every now and then. It was my dope; my way of getting high. If Mom had found my pouch it would have blown her away.

●◇ ◇●

Dear Bud,

I was a young lady when your Yanks marched into the Paris they liberated. We girls thought the handsome Americans were the most exciting men. They were so cute and cleancut. We soon found out just how cleancut they were. I recall being so disappointed that the Yanks didn't smell like men. That wonderful aroma was replaced, frankly, by the stench of stale saliva.

I chose not to follow the Yanks, like the other girls, and married a wonderfully uncircumcised Parisian gentleman. We immigrated to America and had two sons ... who remained French where it counts. I love the aroma of my men.

●◇ ◇●

Dear Bud,

I am a member of my college crew team. Whenever we compete, I try to find the opportunity to sneak back into the locker room, go into lockers of the visiting team, and take a whiff of each man's shorts. That way I can tell just which fellows are uncut.

Dear Bud,

I am an officer in the Navy and was circumcised ten years ago at a special Navy circumcision clinic in San Diego. I was told that my uncircumcised status might hinder my advancement, as I worked with food. I had to wait months for my turn at the clinic, so I suppose they were pretty busy cutting off sailors' skins. Two fellows got it with me, both Latinos, and they were sort of nervous about the whole thing. It didn't bother me at all. They put a curtain up over my chest so I couldn't watch them work on my dick, but I could look sidewise beyond the curtain and I watched both the other fellows get their dicks skinned. I was fascinated. I adjusted to my cut cock quickly and I like it. My only problem is that I miss the smell. My cock just doesn't smell right. It's crazy, but now that my dick doesn't produce cheese anymore, I am hungry for it. I never chased after men in my life until now. Now, all I want is to meet an uncircumcised man who'll let me smell his cheese.

Dear Bud,

I met this great-looking dude who turned on to me when I told him I was uncircumcised. When we got to his place and stripped for action, all he did was sniff. I stood there all evening with an aching boner while he just sniffed at it. Geez, what is wrong with some of these creeps? Does my dick smell any different? I get kind of embarrassed thinking about it.

Dear Bud,

I am uncircumcised and was taught to keep my penis squeaky-clean. I can't stand to let my smegma accumulate and ripen. I have a friend, a married man, who likes me and asks me not to clean my cock for a week before we get together. I hate it, but I know that it means a lot to him. He's circumcised. I understand smegma is the cause of penis cancer. How long is it safe to allow it to ripen?

Dear "Smegma" people,

Smegma, the mysterious white substance that collects under the foreskin, has been accused of many evils: from bad smells to cancer. Webster defines smegma as "the cheesy substance between the glans penis and foreskin (in the male) and around the clitoris and labia minora (in the female)." Many a GI, caught with smegma when ordered to "scat back" during a short-arm inspection, was thus ordered to the circumciser. Many a teenager, who can't shower often enough to keep up with the production of the stuff, has been sent to the family doctor because he "refuses to keep himself clean."

Doctors, parents, coaches, wives, and other sex partners have long thought of smegma as disgusting, smelly dirt. Is smegma dirt? Ask any uncircumcised man who scrubs daily: his smegma is a natural bodily secretion and not the result of his personal neglect. It collects more rapidly at times and production seems to freeze up at other times. Some men produce almost none. Puberty-age boys seem to be the biggest producers, although some older men provide close competition. Different foreskin types seem to produce the stuff at different rates. The survey of young German army recruits, which I mentioned earlier, found smegma on only 12 percent of group B (short foreskins), and 23 percent of group C (long foreskins), 35 percent of group D (tight fore-skins), and 0 percent of group A (no foreskins). They couldn't get inside the penises of group E (phimosed) to determine the presence of smegma.

What did Mother Nature have in mind when she invented smegma? The French know! Connoisseurs of aroma, the French have long used secretions from the genitals of male animals as the base for some of their most expensive per-fumes. The most popular scents are musk (the smegma of the musk-ox); civet (from the sex organs of the African civet cat); and castor (from the genital glands of the beaver). Chuck Daniels, an expert on the production of fragrances, wrote about this in the second issue of the *Uncut America Newsletter*. He hid in the haylofts above the cages of animals at various French perfume factories as he watched the workers annoy the animals "until they fell down in their cages frothing at the mouth and gaping for air."

"As I lay there in the straw," he wrote,

I watched these men gleefully and with much joking and rubbing at their crotches proceed to scrape out ... a special male pouch just above the anus of the wild cheetah. The unforgettable raw odor certainly excited me as it wafted up in the loft. The animals were regularly tormented each day, I later learned, to activate their valuable male gland, which corresponds in man to the glans-penis and to the prepuce of the musk-ox.

If the scent of a musk-ox's smegma is so prized, why then is human smegma so despised? Olfactory reaction to scent is a subjective, learned experience. Soft-ripened cheeses are not everybody's favorite smell, nor is human "musk." But obviously, judging from the letters I've received, the odor of the uncircumcised penis has its devotees. That they include circumcised men might be explained in a report of a scientific study reported in *CoEvolution Quarterly*. The author found that intermale aggression among mice is controlled by pheromones produced by the foreskin. Circumcised mice were more aggressive, apparently because their uncircumcised companions released pheromones that stimulated aggressive behavior from the circumcised animals. Dr. Robert Da Prato, reporting on this study, posed the following question: "Since the human prepuce produces numerous odoriferous complex chemicals, is it possible that this mechanism is operating to some extent in humans?"[3]

Much of the prejudice against smegma originated with reports that it can cause penile cancer. With the invention of soap, that stopped needing to be a concern. Even under adverse conditions of war, a man can swab out his foreskin with saliva.

Smegma, which curdles and hardens under the foreskin, certainly can irritate the sensitive inner mucosa. While most doctors report that regular bathing habits are the best way to avoid foreskin problems, many report that it is not necessary to "scat back" every time you shower. Every few days is enough. Scrubbing it out after sex is a hygienic plus. However, the secret of pleasing the devotees of "musk" while keeping yourself clean as well is to use pure soap, not antibacterial deodorant soaps. That should keep you safely clean ... and your hot dates happy!

Dear Bud,

Where in hell did the term "lace curtains" come from? I am every inch (7 $\frac{1}{2}$ of them) a man and that includes my foreskin. I resent people calling my foreskin "lace curtains" because it sounds so feminine. How could a part of the penis be referred to in feminine terms? Sure, some guys might be effeminate, but as long as they have a cock swinging between their legs they are men.

Maleskin

Dear Maleskin,

I agree. It boggles the mind to think an effeminate term can be applied to the penis. However, "lace curtains" has been commonly used in reference to the foreskin for a hundred years. Another derogatory term is "ruffled foreskin" or "rumpled foreskin." The words "lace" and "ruffled" are the keys to answer your question. It all started in Victorian England when ruffles, frills, and lace were fashionable in male attire. English gentlemen wore lace and they certainly didn't consider it effeminate.

Ruffled curtains adorned every window in Victorian London. As they were hung in a huge flurry of lace, they came to be called "lace curtains." Well, as the gentleman's prepuce also hung in a flurry of ruffles, it too became known, affectionately, as "lace curtains."

Not until this century did the derogatory term "rumple-foreskin" came into general use. I suppose after they chopped off most of London's foreskins, the few remaining ones were an unfamiliar, "ugly" sight. As the last generation of uncircumcised men aged, the younger circumcised generation referred to the old men as "Rumpleforeskin." Thankfully, with more and more foreskins popping into familiar view, "Rumpleforeskin" is disappearing.

While we're at it, let's have some fun and review the synonyms that have been used through the centuries for the foreskin:

anteater	cock warmer	Greek's pride
army flaps	covering	Hollywood shades
case	curtains	hood
cavalier	flagsheath	Junior's aimer
cock cozy	grandpa's flag	lace curtains

love curtains	pouch	shades
man's pride	pumper	skinhead
manskin	Robin Hood	snapper
manwrapper	roll	St. Paul's medal
meat casing	Roman shades	wad
monk's hood	rose bud	wad of fat
old soldier's flag	rosette	wing flaps
pillcock	sexskin	wrapper
pointer	sextube	

P.S. The current favored words for the uncircumcised penis: *whole* and *natural*.

Dear Bud,

My curiosity about the uncircumcised penis is relentless. Although I am a married heterosexual, I have stood at public urinals trying to sneak a glimpse at an uncut man pissing. Never having a foreskin of my own, I can't figure out how the stream passes through that skin and maintains a steady stream. Why doesn't it just dribble out? I have surmised that some men pull their foreskin back off their urethral opening, but I have seen many who just let the skin flop where it may. Can you explain the technique of urinating with a foreskin?

Relentless

Dear Relentless,

I admit that urinating "through that skin" must be learned; it isn't as easy as using a circumcised "aimer." One thing that really angers the mothers of uncut boys is the mess they make in the bathroom while they learn how to use "one of those things." Actually, urinating is one of the activities, besides masturbation, that naturally loosens up a growing boy's foreskin.

To answer your question, Relentless, let's review another letter received by the USA:

I have a favorite peephole, viewing two urinals in a men's room at the university at which I work. My hobby is watching uncircumcised men piss. The endless variety of methods keeps me fascinated. Of course, out of every 100 pissing peters at the school, only about 15 have foreskin. I am interested only in those 15. So, here are my findings:

- 5 of the 15 roll their skins all the way back, completely clearing their glans while pissing.
- 5 of the 15 roll their skin back just enough to clear the stream or slightly further.
- 3 don't touch their foreskins and merely allow the stream to splash awkwardly through the skin funnel. One of these usually pulls out his balls while he pisses.
- 1 pinches his foreskin shut while the stream builds up inside and then lets it out with a swoosh. Then he pinches again, builds it up again and swoosh. He repeats the process several times.

When they are done:

- Then, 6 out of the first 10 carefully pull their skins forward, giving them a tug at the tip, and then put them snugly away.
- 4 of the first 10 merely shove their cocks in their pants with their skins still retracted at various positions.
- 2 of the next 3 shake their penis violently, pulling their foreskin back and forward several times, clearing out any trapped urine.
- 1 of those three now pulls his skin all the way back and wipes his bared cockhead dry with his shirttail.
- The pincher, after a long suspenseful wait for another swoosh which doesn't come, lets his foreskin fall shut with an audible snap and flips it into his pants.

Oh yes, the 15th pisser. He spreads his forward-position foreskin open with two fingers so that the glans never shows but his stream neatly clears the skin with an unobstructed path. When he is finished, he keeps his foreskin spread wide with his fingers, pulls his penis up to his stomach, bends over and looks inside it. Then, having a second thought, he suddenly looks around the room suspecting that someone is watching. I quickly move away from the peephole and record my findings for the day.

Dear Bud,

Here are my statistics: Born in 1960, New England, Scottish descent, straight and never had sex with a male but am bisexual in my fantasies. I would love to share my foreskin someday with a man who doesn't have one of his own, as long as it is done discreetly.

I have noticed in the locker room of my country club my very macho friends seem to go bland and stare glaze-eyed at my genitals. Until I read your book [*Foreskin*, first edition] it never occurred to me that these fellows might just be painfully curious about the foreskin which they never had. I sometimes feel embarrassed or odd, but I love the visual attention and wish my friends had the balls to back up their stares with a question about my cock, or even a physical approach. But, hell, all I do is stare myself ... guess I am 99% heterosexual. I am a good-looking young guy, sort of the executive type, and am in great shape. Do you think any of your USA members would like to give my foreskin a look-over? Maybe one of them will teach me how to "dock" my skin over a circumcised cock, so I'll know how to share it with another male?

Country Clubber

Dear Sir!

The 10-inch Marine dick I carry between my legs is uncut as hell! It's got so much fuckin' skin on it, it droops a good two inches off the end of my pisshole. It doesn't even come to a tip, it just flops wide open. In fact, all you have to do is lift up my dick and look inside the skin and, even without a scat-back, you get a good view of what's going on in there. Even with all that skin, my whole works are in plain view. I hang out at this beer joint near the base and the fuckers all line up in the raunchy latrine and take turns poking their cut dicks into my wad. Hell, I can cover two dicks at once!

Now, here's my secret. I widen my foreskin with bottle caps or caps off toothpaste tubes, etc. I scat back and push the cap against my pisshole. Then I bring the roll back up and trap the cap inside. I pick caps which are wider around than my stiff dick. This keeps my skin so fuckin' wide that it can take any size Marine shaft that comes along.

At Attention!

Dear Bud,

My foreskin is long, tapered, and overhangs longer than most other skins I've seen. Now that foreskin is popular I have all these cut dudes wanting to know how my skin would feel over their naked dicks. We poke at it, try stretching it out wide, twist, yank, and pull at my foreskin but my cock just won't allow another cock to get inside. I can't figure it out. My skin is loose enough. How do you dock penises?

Stubborn Penis

Dear Docking People,

"Docking" is the current popular term for the coming together of two penises, like the coming together of two space capsules. Right now, the most popular "docking" experience is for an uncircumcised man to pull his foreskin over the glans of a circumcised man. Yes, it is usually possible. The USA has received hundreds of letters asking about the safety of docking. Is it safe sex? Who knows? If the penis has no sores and ejaculation doesn't take place, I don't see how there could be any significant risk. However, I believe you should be honest about your HIV status with a partner before any sexual contact takes place. Now, in answer to the above dockers:

First, Country Clubber. It's amazing how many circumcised heterosexual men are curious about foreskin. It's generally the only interest they have in their own gender. The USA files are full of letters from such men. After a close inspection, watching the skin roll over the glans, most of these men are satisfied. However, once the realization that it is possible for an uncircumcised man to place his foreskin over the glans of a circumcised penis, a mere visual "look-over" may no longer suffice ... even for your macho friends.

Second, the Marine. Did you say ten inches of Marine dick? Gulp! Oh, pardon me. Back to your letter. Thanks for your widening technique. You've got one healthy roll on that Marine dick, mister! I'm sure it can take anything that comes along. However, I'd advise readers to be careful of both abrasiveness and toxic matter when using bottle caps. Otherwise, I think your stretching method is great.

Third, Stubborn Penis. The key to your problem is that your foreskin is tapered. I'll bet your skin even stays forward

135

when you get erect. Right? Tapered foreskins usually have weighted tips. That is, the skin around the tip is thicker than the foreskin that covers the glans. It appears to be "pouted." It is the weighted tip, which may seem like a tiny circular muscle, that keeps the foreskin full-forward over an erection.

Stubborn, your foreskin will never be easily docked. You can stretch it, but that will only make it longer and bulkier and that stubborn ring of foreskin tip will not yield much width. Count yourself lucky, my friend, because that weighted tip is an extra bonus that nature gave you, and it feels sensational as it stretches over your glans. That little ring gives your penis a particularly effective massage, a sensation unknown by most men. It's almost like a rubber band dancing up and down and around your manhood. But, dancing over someone else's "manhood" won't be easy for you. I would suggest, before attempting to dock, that you soak your penis in warm, soapless water. Dry it completely, then stretch your foreskin over the intended recipient before erections occur. It will be a struggle to keep everything in place as the penises rise to the occasion but well worth the effort if you make a circumcised man happy. Share your good fortune.

Dear Bud,

Whenever I retract my foreskin for any reason, then allow it to roll back over my glans by itself, it doesn't make it all the way. The tip folds under the skin and leaves a small part of the glans exposed. Leaving it folded under can be irritating, especially around my pisshole. I must actually stop whatever I'm doing, go somewhere private, pull out my dick, and tug my foreskin tip out of its trap. Do other uncircumcised men report this problem?

Trapped Tip

Dear Trapped Tip,

Yes, as a matter of fact, this very intimate, personal adjustment is one that most uncircumcised men must make several times a day. The weighted foreskin tip does fold under the foreskin as it rolls forward over the glans, often leaving the meatus exposed. With the thumb and index

After the adjustment

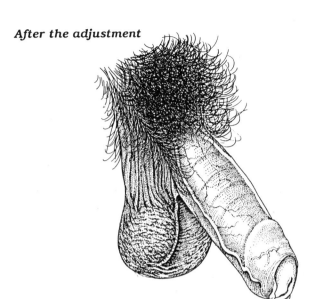

finger, a slight tug at the bottom lip of the foreskin is generally adequate to bring the tip out to its natural pointed position.

Most men do this so automatically they'd be surprised the adjustment is even mentioned in a book. But for readers to whom the foreskin is a stranger, this bit of trivia may be considered a contribution to their education. The next time you observe an uncut man or boy giving himself a tug, you'll know what's going on.

●◇ ◇●

Dear Bud,

I read about the frenum in your book but I can't figure out what it is. Where is it on my cock? I'm cut, by the way.

Dear Cut,

The frenum, or frenulum, according to Webster's dictionary is "a connecting fold of membrane to support or restrain a part of the anatomy (as the tongue)." Feel under your tongue. Do you notice that strip of skin stretching vertically under it? Now, lift up your cock and look under the head, at the point where the two parts come together like a valentine.

The frenum on a circumcised penis

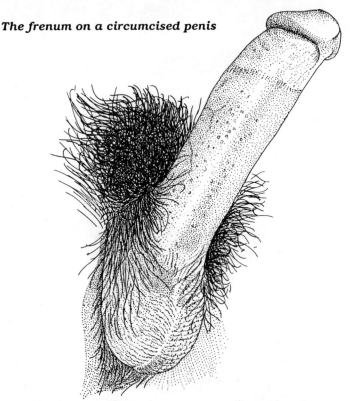

Do you see a tiny piece of skin stretched vertically there? If so, that is your frenum. Some circumcisers carve it away along with the foreskin so I can't guarantee you'll find one on your circumcised penis. You will find a frenum on most uncircumcised penises and many circumcised ones. In fact, many cut men claim their frenum to be their most sensitive part. What is the natural function of the frenum? It's nature's way of keeping the foreskin forward. Otherwise, like the tongue without its frenulum, the foreskin would probably roll back. Yes, nature wants the foreskin to remain forward.

●◇ ◇●

Dear Bud,

I dig mutual jack-off sessions and especially enjoy it with fellow uncuts. The visual aspects are heightened by watching foreskin roll back and forth over the cockhead. However,

I've noticed that most uncuts never use lubricants. I always put Vaseline on my glans before sexual activity. I suppose it's because my mother made me put Vaseline on my penis when I was a boy (though I can't remember why). I don't get off as well without a lubricant, but I wonder if the habit interferes with my penile sensitivity. Do you think lubricants disturb the natural sensitivity I would have with an unlubricated foreskin rolling over an unlubricated glans? I would love to have sex without sticky hands.

Sticky Hands

Dear Sticky Hands,

It's true that most uncircumcised men have an advantage in that they don't have to use lubricants. Lube manufacturers owe the nation's circumcisers a huge debt. Some uncircumcised men do have drier glans and drier-textured foreskin than others and must use lubricants to avoid abrasion.

Your preference for lubricants may stem from these factors, or it may be more related to your childhood use of Vaseline. (Your mother probably heard Vaseline recommended to keep your skin from "sticking.") Whatever the reason, it certainly does no harm, and if it enhances your sexual enjoyment, then my advice is to keep using it.

NOTES

1. Robert Chartham, Ph.D., *Advice to Men* (London: Tandem Publishing, 1971), p. 90.

2. Eichelschutz Hautlob, in "Clothing and the Foreskin," *Clothes Dick*, Vol. 2, No. 2.

3. Dr. Robert A. Da Prato in the *Medical Journal of Australia*, Sept. 29, 1984, p. 479. The study he refers to was reported by S. Garden, "Of Circumcised Mice and Men," in *CoEvolution Quarterly*, 1981, p. 107.

2. Options, Opinions

*D*ear Bud,

I graduated from high school when I was eighteen. The Vietnam War was going on and I was a patriotic kid, so I joined the Navy. After boot camp at San Diego, instead of Vietnam I was assigned to the H.Q. of the 6th Fleet at Naples. We had routine short-arm inspections every few weeks. If you're interested in cocks this is a real experience because the doctor had everyone milk them [that is, pull on it rhythmically, as if milking a cow]. The 10 percent or so who were not cut had to peel back their foreskins and bare the head, as well as go through the milking routine. I never had any trouble at these inspections until a new doctor showed up. He seemed particularly interested in my cock and made me skin it several times.

I knew I always had a long foreskin, but I didn't think there was anything physically wrong with it. When my cock was soft the skin hung about an inch beyond the head and was longer in back than front. The skin was pretty thick and somewhat tight, but I could always pull it back when my prick was soft. When I pissed I peeled the skin back every time so that no piss ran through the foreskin. I always kept my cock clean, tugging the skin back every time I showered and then soaping my penis thoroughly, then pulling the skin out again. This was a real sensual experience. Sometimes when I couldn't get a shower every day some smelly gunk would form but that wasn't very often. The next shower would take care of that. Most of my buddies were cut and I often thought how much they were missing by not having a long, moist foreskin like mine.

However, my foreskin was too tight to pull back when I had a hard-on. I've got about 7 1/2 inches hard and pretty thick. When it stiffened up there would be still about half an inch of skin hanging tight beyond the tip of the head. No matter how hard I pulled on it, the opening was too small to let the head pop out. This never bothered me because there was still plenty of play in the whole shaft and the head felt good moving back and forth inside the skin. When I shot maybe it wasn't as direct as other guys but still it spurted from the folds of the skin. I jacked off at least once a day. Sometimes I would pinch the end tight together with my left hand and beat off with my right until the jism shot and sloshed around the head. Man, what a feeling! Nobody I ever had sex with complained about my long foreskin and a lot of my buddies told me it really turned them on. In spite of all that crap about "cut is cleaner," I think they envied the long sheath over the end of my cock. Now that I'm cut, every time I see a natural cock I know just how they feel.

Anyway, getting back to the doctor. I reported to him in sick bay. He had me skin it back again and sort of clucked when he saw all the folds of skin piled up behind the head. Then he had me pull the skin out again and he measured the length of my foreskin. He wanted me to get a hard-on and left so I could get it up in private. This was a tough job but I thought about my last liberty, so when he came back my dick was ready for him. He tugged and pulled on the skin but as usual it stayed bunched together beyond the damned head. I think the creep just hated guys who had not been cut as babies or maybe he was some kind of kooky closet queen who was envious of me. Anyway, he said I had to report for a circumcision. He blew my mind! I told him I never had any VD, I never had trouble cleaning myself, and I never had any problem with shooting off. I told him I didn't want to go around minus my foreskin and with a scar ringing around my dick. I told him, "I'll be damned if I'm going to report!" You know what that motherfucker said to me next? "Okay, sailor, then it's a court-martial or a general discharge for you." Well, I didn't want that on my record and I knew I couldn't beat the system.

So now I have a cock just like all the other poor bastards whose folks didn't have enough sense to say "No Way!" when the doctor asked if they wanted to have the baby cut. I can tell you the Navy took away a lot of sensual pleasure when they mutilated me. I sure miss my long, slithery foreskin. Now that it's gone, fucking and jacking off is like doing it with a dry pole. Someday the men of this country will put an end to all this crazy cock-cutting and their dicks will be like nature made them and like mine used to be.

Chopped against My Will

●◇ ◇●

Dear Bud,

While in the Army I was stationed at a military hospital in Honolulu. It seemed that every serviceman in Hawaii was coming in to get circumcised, especially the sailors. They roamed the hospital with their little cans of anesthetic spray. I kept asking why they had it done and the answers boiled down to the fact they had been told all the nourishment needed to feed that extra skin would now be used to make their cocks double or triple in size and increase the size of their cockheads. Wouldn't you want to be circumcised if that was true? I didn't believe a word of it and still have my skin and my cock sure isn't puny, either! Those poor stupid bastards don't know what they've missed ... or maybe they do?

Still Intact

●◇ ◇●

Dear Bud,

I thought I would share with your readers some of my observations from my stay in the U.S. Navy. I was a commissary in the supply department on a ship, and in 1968 we left San Diego for a tour of the Far East. We encountered a typhoon and spent longer at sea than scheduled, and everyone got bored as hell. One particular hospital corpsman aboard the ship became quite friendly with supply department personnel. He would hang around and shoot the breeze, I suppose hoping to get special favors from us in the way of food and supplies.

One day he strolled in with his green surgical garb. He complained that he had to work all alone that day because the young apprentice corpsman just assigned to him was so fidgety while he was performing circumcisions that he told the kid to leave the room. We were all sort of shocked and embarrassed at his doing circumcisions and when we questioned him about it, he said that he'd already gone through most of the foreskins aboard the ship and was to receive a special letter of praise from his superior officer for performing the circumcisions. I spoke up and asked if he really felt all those circumcisions were necessary and he said that all he cared was that the men had requested them and he was merely giving them what they wanted. He went on to say that he "didn't mind" circumcising a dick because there wasn't much else to do on the ship anyway.

I later found out that this corpsman was, himself, still uncircumcised. I have no doubt that by the time we arrived in the Philippines his was the last foreskin on the ship. Bud, I was circumcised at birth and have always resented the fact. I'm not gay, but have often wondered about those men who got trimmed in the military. What did they think about their new circumcised penis once they returned to their wives and girlfriends ... or boyfriends, for that matter?

I'm not fooled when I hear that someone "volunteered" for something in the Navy. I believe that if enough ex-military people who were pressured into circumcision would come forward, we could bring a class-action suit against the government. Maybe we could halt these unnecessary mutilations, and bring an end to forced circumcision in our country. I don't know about the present military, but I know from personal experience that many GIs returned home without the foreskin they had when they joined up. Let me know your thoughts on this. I remain fighting mad.

Fighting Mad

Dear "Ex-Military" People,

In our history of foreskin, we read how the growth of the military in this country seemed to parallel the growth of circumcision. Many anthropologists theorize that it is the warrior tribes, or their warrior classes, who are most prone to circumcision among the primitives. It's difficult to apply such a theory to developed societies, especially when you consider the uncircumcised Spartans or Nazis. Still, the badge of manhood seems to translate into circumcision in many all-male situations.

A class-action lawsuit, such as you describe, has been discussed in anti-circumcision circles for years. However, the statute of limitations pretty well wipes out the possibility of such action for most men circumcised during their service. What we need is a fresh, young, apple-faced recruit who recently lost his foreskin to the whim of a corpsman. But you and I both know that such a kid is much too shy about his penis to discuss it before a jury. After all, he was probably too embarrassed even to defend his foreskin in the military and most probably signed the "voluntary" circumcision release. After all, his current training has him accepting authority without question. "Yessir! Sircumcise it, sir!"

Fortunately, things are changing in the new, professional military. The services have drastically reduced their medical corps. One USA member, now in the Navy, claims that medical records no longer indicate the circumcision status of naval personnel. In 1985, the Army even halted infant circumcision at two of its hospitals in Germany. Lieutenant General Quinn H. Becker, the Army Surgeon, claimed "this age-old procedure serves no medical benefit and poses a small risk." Opposition to his order came from the soldiers and their wives who demanded that their sons be circumcised. Becker advised, "My objective is to educate people so they can make a totally rational decision and not an emotional decision or one based only on what's been done in the past."

Actually, Mad, I don't believe that any branch of the armed forces ever had a circumcision requirement. The procedure was usually left to the decision of individual medics, or the chief medical officer of a post. After all, their job was to keep the men healthy and ready for combat action. There are stories from the various wars about how nonmedical officers preferred to have their men circumcised, and it seems that most medics were only too willing to cooperate. All you have to do is to dig through the old World War II military medical bulletins and find many "how to" articles: how to do quick circumcisions, how to circumcise without a general anesthesia (in order to get the man back in action quick), how to convince a man he should be circumcised, and so on. The Navy even used a "one-size-fits-all" adult circumcision tool patented in the early forties. Most of the medics were drafted right out of medical school, or were being educated by the military, and one of their first lessons told them that circumcision prevented VD, cancer, and masturbation. There is no doubt that many men "volunteered" for circumcision; some for valid medical reasons.

What happens to men in all-male situations? Why are they so anxious to circumcise or be circumcised? Here are three episodes, reported to the USA, that might give us some insight:

• I was a medic, just out of school, stationed in postwar South Korea during the '60s. Each post, scattered throughout the area, had at least one medic. We took turns spending one week away from our posts to inspect all the incoming personnel disembarking at the main port. After the short-arm inspection, we secretly made up a list of all the incoming uncircumcised men, and circulated it around the medical post. This was to alert our fellow medics that "there was something to do." Without a war going on, and with a huge, idle army, we were simply bored to death. One medic at a remote installation begged us to send him one of the men on the uncut list. As the foreskins fell, subsequent lists were circulated indicating which man had been successfully circumcised. Then a new list of arriving recruits would come just in time to make life interesting again.

• I was a naval medic during my tour of Vietnam. I promoted circumcision with every opportunity. If a patient resisted, I merely gave him a physical examination, which included a little rough handling of his penis to the point of its erection. I usually got my circumcision release signed. Then, without seeking it, I had my first homosexual experience. I immediately took stock of myself and my motives and quit the Navy. I admitted to myself that I was circumcising those fellows just as an excuse to get my hands on their genitals. I am now in private practice and refuse to circumcise any patient.

• Twenty years ago I was in Vietnam as a 19-year-old draftee. I was assigned to an officer who was an attaché to a general. We lived together in a bungalow in Saigon and we traveled extensively with the general. At first, I was terrified by the shells and bombs that we heard from our bungalow and would lay in bed and literally shake. The officer felt sorry for me and occasionally got in my bed during the air raids to calm me down. I wasn't gay at the time, or at least I didn't know anything about being gay, but when he cuddled me it sure helped. Then one day I got word that my grandfather had died and I couldn't help but cry. Again, he cuddled me and that night he brought me out. I was in love. After a few weeks though, I noticed he became hesitant and I figured it was because I was uncircumcised. He was cut. We had a friend who was a medical officer and who was also gay. I went to his office one afternoon to ask him to circumcise me. He was away on a mission so another medic inspected my penis and agreed to circumcise it right there on the spot. For some stupid reason I got an erection. He told me to get it soft. The harder I tried to get my damned penis flaccid, the more erect it got. Finally he told me to go home and get some sex and return the next day. When I got home I got orders to travel, so it was a few days before I could return to the clinic. I didn't say a word about my pending circumcision to my lover. Our gay friend was back in his office when I showed up for it and he gave me hell! "Leave that foreskin alone!" he shouted. "You're lucky, kid. Most of the medics around here would love to get their knives on your dick! Go home." I walked home dejected, not knowing that our friend was phoning my lover. When I got home, my lover asked me where I had been. I tried to lie but the truth came out. He said, "I admit that I was confused by your foreskin. C'mon, let's get in bed and educate ourselves." He was my first love … he was killed by a bomb.

●◇ ◇●

Dear Bud,

How in hell did some Americans escape the knife? Fore-skins were few and far between among my peers in Houston. I would like to know just how some babies lucked out? I have posed the question to the few uncut adults I have met and, damn, they don't know the answer. Do you?

Unlucky in Houston

●◇ ◇●

Dear Houston,

It is true that most uncut men have no idea how they "lucked out." But from what I have gleaned from medical professionals and parents, the following are the most frequent causes of American noncircumcision:

1. Premature birth. Premature infants are seldom circumcised at birth.
2. Immigrant parents. Infants born to foreign-born immigrants have a better chance of keeping their foreskin than those born to later-generation American parents.
3. Hemophilia. Hemophiliacs cannot be circumcised at birth. During the seventies, Israeli doctors began circumcising older hemophiliacs by using a laser beam, a procedure that reduces the risk of bleeding.
4. Father's decision. The father wanted his son to "look like" him: uncircumcised. Or the father was circumcised and resented it.
5. Older brother died, or was injured, during his circumcision. Yes, sadly, this tragic reason is the one given by several USA members. Their parents weren't about to go through that trauma with subsequent sons.
6. Born in a rural area. Old country doctors seemed to be the last to jump on the circumcision bandwagon. "The doctor didn't believe in it," many a farm boy told the USA. Most of these fellows were born in their homes, where circumcision tools weren't handy. Unfortunately, the old family doctor seems to have gone into history in many rural areas.

So, if you are wondering about a guy but are afraid to ask, just ask him if he was born premature, or on a farm. "Preemies" often grow up to be big sturdy hunks ... and we all know about farm boys.

●◇ ◇●

Dear Bud,

At the age of eight, I was the only boy I knew who hadn't been circumcised — my father failed to pay my delivery fee on time, so the obstetrician refused to do it to me. I had no trouble being uncircumcised until high school, when I came down with a case of venereal warts. I have many veins on the surface of my penis, more than I have observed on any other male. The foreskin had two veins in it the size of a pencil, with smaller veins branching off the two larger veins. The foreskin, itself, was rather thin and delicate, making the veins appear very prominent.

When I developed the warts, my frenulum and sur-rounding foreskin became very swollen, making me unwill-ing to retract the skin. It didn't interfere with urination. The doctor treating my warts wanted to circumcise me but my parents couldn't afford it. The warts disappeared until I was twenty-eight, when they returned. My doctor told me that a pliable, delicate foreskin and frenulum like mine will never have a permanent phimosis because it was so easily stretched, but that same pliability allows small tears to develop during intercourse which made me susceptible to the virus that causes warts. So, two years ago I was circumcised.

I'll never forget masturbating the night before surgery. The soft skin rolling back and forth over my sensitive glans felt wonderful; my orgasm was extremely intense. I studied my foreskin for the last time. Its veins were engorged and seemed to enhance my manhood, and both my foreskin and glans were vivid pink, which was erotic just to ob-serve. Best of all, I could feel the sensitive folds of skin which always gave me pleasure during intercourse. The next day, I watched my circumcision from beginning to end — an erotic, unforgettable experience in itself!

Now my penis is much less sensitive and the head has turned a dull gray color. I miss those folds of skin during intercourse. But, to climax my story, the venereal warts returned. Now I wish I had left well-enough alone. Can you ask your urologists in the USA this question for me ... to get rid of my warts what's next — cutting off my cock?

Circumcised

Dear Circumcised,

I can understand your disappointment at losing your beloved foreskin for naught. To retrieve your faith in urology, and hoping that you will not have to lose any more of your manhood, I have indeed consulted Dr. Skinnon, my USA urologist consultant:

> I'm glad you got to watch your circumcision and found it to be "erotic and unforgettable" because that is the only good you got out of it. Warts are viral in origin, as you describe, but they are usually self-limiting, meaning they come and go whenever they are good and ready. This happened to you after the high school experience and you were spared their reappearance until age twenty-eight. They continue to come and go on susceptible individuals with or without foreskin. Treatment by local application or removal of the warts themselves would have been my choice of therapy and you could have left your delicate foreskin intact. Some warts are large and ugly. If they appear to be coming out of the pisshole they are potentially dangerous and require immediate urological attention. However, (as a urologist) I only circumcise a patient if he feels his foreskin interferes with his ability to attract partners and I must be pretty convinced of his problems before he can buy it from me.

Well, Circumcised, all I can say to you, and others who have foreskin problems, is to shop around for urologists. When the verdict is circumcision, get a second opinion. Anyway, you sound like a sexy guy and I'm sure you are enjoying what you have left.

●◇ ◇●

Dear Bud,

I am a female nurse. I think your writings minimize the medical reasons for circumcision too much. They also emphasize the discomfort infants suffer during circumcision. I have witnessed over 300 circumcisions and about half the babies slept through it. I have also cared for patients with cancer of the penis who needed their penis surgically removed. They go through a very traumatic experience as do their families.

Interested Nurse

Dear Nurse,

Thanks for your observations. Yes, my writings are meant to emphasize the social, emotional, and erotic aspects of circumcision. The medical aspects are well known to many Americans and easily available. This book is not a medical book. I always advise my correspondents who have a medical problem to visit a urologist. I have no intention of giving a diagnosis.

When we discuss routine infant circumcision as preventive medicine, however, let us recall the attendant risks. In the year 1962, when circumcision was practically universal in the U.S., there were 232 deaths nationwide from penile cancer while, during the same year, approximately 153 deaths resulted from infant circumcision. Hardly a fair trade-off. While I'm not a doctor, I do know something of male anatomy. Several types of vital sensory nerve receptors get lopped off as your sleeping baby boys are circumcised. I can understand your interest in circumcision as preventive medicine, but have you ever considered the erotic pleasures a foreskin can give a man and his partner?

One more point of controversy must be addressed, Nurse, and that is your statement that "half the babies slept through it." Anti-circumcisionists insist that the operation causes a momentary, and possibly long-lasting, pain to all babies; pro-circumcisionists insist that it doesn't hurt them. Fran Porter, a research associate in pediatrics at St. Louis Children's Hospital, has concluded that "there's absolutely no evidence to support the notion that infants don't feel pain ... and now we have evidence that refutes that idea." She states that the cries of newborn boys being circumcised without anesthesia changed in dramatic ways — their cries became shorter, more rapid, and more frantic.[1] According to pediatrician Adrian MacFarlane, "After a newborn baby has been circumcised, his sleep patterns are disturbed ... It is possible that some reported differences in behavior between male and female babies are results of [circumcision] instead of any innate differences."[2]

●◇ ◇●

Dear Bud,

I thought you might find this *disgusting* article, which

appeared in the August 15, 1989, issue of the *Boston Globe*, of interest:

> The foreskins removed from babies during circumcision are ideal skin grafts for elderly people, diabetics, paraplegics and others suffering from chronic skin ulcers, according to Boston University and Harvard researchers, whose report appears in this month's *Journal of American Academy of Dermatology* ... Cultured grafts derived from neonatal foreskin offer the advantages of rapid growth in culture and immediate availability, concluded Dr. Tanis Phillips of Boston University.

Disgusted

Dear Disgusted,

Infant foreskin has long been prized as healthy human tissue for use in scientific exploration. Several years ago when it was thought that the new drug interferon was the miracle that might stop cancer, it was reported that foreskin fiberblasts were used in its manufacture. Word got out that a huge foreskin "harvest" was about to commence. Some members of the Uncircumcised Society of America quickly requested that their names be dropped from our roster and took their foreskins into hiding. We had visions of "foreskin banks" where we would be paid for our circumcisions. Just how many foreskins were they going to need?

A prominent physician in Seattle, a USA supporter, investigated the worrisome situation and wrote,

> Don't lose sleep over it. The plant in Virginia [producing interferon] already has its cell lines or stocks, and as a guess maybe twenty-five foreskins would be used. You can get tons of interferon from one foreskin, and the line could be used for years. So, one foreskin could keep a lot of people busy indefinitely. Fiberblasts can be obtained from other tissue but foreskins are more readily available than, say, ears.

Thanks, Doc.

Dear Bud,

I am uncircumcised and I worry about reports that I

may be exposed to more diseases because of the presence of my foreskin. What are the current medical reasons for circumcision?

Should I Worry?

Dear Worry,

Let's go to one of the nation's authorities on circumcision, Aaron Fink, M.D., who writes:

> In addition to the fact that [circumcision] facilitates penile hygiene, a daily requirement for uncircumcised males, it has been shown to have several benefits including the following points.
> • Recent studies have shown that routine neonatal circumcision decreases the incidence of urinary tract infections from 10- to 20-fold.
> • Several studies have pointed to a decrease in the incidence of sexually transmitted diseases among circumcised men.
> • Newborn circumcision virtually eliminates the risk of penile cancer.
> • It also eliminates phimosis and paraphimosis.
> • Evidence is mounting that there may be a connection of papilloma virus with penile cancer and cervical cancer. Studies have shown that the same virus types are implicated in both; thus the hypothesis is that it's possible to transmit the virus through intercourse.[3]

As readers know by now, the medical community is far from unified behind Dr. Fink's arguments. The important point is that any uncircumcised man, or prospective parent, should be well informed on the pros and cons of circumcision before making the big decision. Worry, I suggest you consult your urologist, and then get a second opinion. Dr. Fink concludes his article, "I am not urging or even encouraging that all uncircumcised adult men rush out to have a preventive circumcision. But for the newborn male, it's a different matter. In deciding whether to have a son circumcised, parents will make a decision that may be of great consequence throughout his entire life."

Bouncing back to the opposing school in the circumcision controversy among the medical community, let's review the conclusions of the American Academy of Pediatrics

Committee on the Fetus and Newborn Report of the Ad Hoc Task Force on Circumcision filed in 1975:

1. Prevention of phimosis is not an indication for routine neonatal circumcision because complete separation of the glans and prepuce has not occurred.
2. If neonatal circumcision is not elected, measures for penile hygiene should be outlined for the parents before the birth of the child.
3. Carcinoma of the penis can largely be prevented by circumcision. However, this cancer is rare and good principles of penile hygiene are adequate prophylactic alternatives.
4. Circumcision does not decrease the risk of cancer of the prostate.
5. Incidence of carcinoma of the cervix is not decreased in sexual partners of circumcised men.
6. Balanitis occurs only in uncircumcised men.
7. There is no evidence that circumcision decreases venereal disease.
8. Circumcision injuries and complications do occur and are not rare.
9. Circumcision may lead to meatal stenosis.
10. Circumcision should not be performed on premature or sick infants, on any subject 12 to 24 hours of age, or any infants with congenital anomaly.
11. Conclusion: There is no absolute medical indication for routine circumcision of the newborn. Therefore, circumcision of the male neonate cannot be considered an essential component of adequate total health care.[4]

Dear Bud,

I was very disturbed by reading about the uncircumcised men in Kenya being more prone to AIDS than their circumcised brothers. But you claim that most men in Kenya are circumcised except for those nontribal men who live in poverty. Can you illuminate?

Disturbed

Dear Disturbed,

AIDS is too serious for anyone to toss around unfounded, or inadequately tested, theories. I do not want to make light of any medical research in the fight against the terrible disease. However, in answer to your question, it is true that most men in Kenya are circumcised and the nation has one of the worst epidemics of AIDS among heterosexuals. Circumcision in that East African nation comes from a convergence of three traditions: (1) the Colonial English; (2) Islam; and (3) the puberty rites of most native African tribes. To illustrate the pervasiveness of circumcision in Kenya, and the fact that some nontribal blacks have escaped it, let's quote a news article reported in Australian newspapers in 1985. According to the *Melbourne Gazette*:

> Two porters in Nairobi's main market were forced by co-workers to undergo circumcision, *The Standard* newspaper reported today. The operation is traditionally carried out on youths in Kenya to mark their coming to manhood. Six additional porters are due to be circumcised on Sunday, the paper said, quoting co-workers as explaining that yesterday's "swoop" was part of an effort to ensure that all porters at Walulima market are circumcised.
>
> The circumcisions, carried out by a doctor at a clinic to which the two were taken in a truck, were deemed necessary because the men, aged 24 and 32, were thought not to have been 'mature' in their behavior, the paper said. A collection was made to pay the doctor for performing the operation. A crowd of 300 market workers, including women, accompanied the two in the truck or followed in other vehicles chanting initiation songs, the report said. After the operation the two were escorted to a place of rest. Male circumcision is obligatory for the Kikuyu and Masai tribes in Kenya. The two men forcibly circumcised yesterday are both believed to be Kikuyu.

Circumcision is prevalent along the eastern coast of Africa. North Africa, being predominantly Moslem, is almost totally circumcised. In the sub-Sahara nations of West Africa and Central Africa, however, large groups of uncircumcised men can be found. These nations retain some of the French-Catholic and Belgian-Catholic influence of their colonial history, when brutal tribal circumcision was discouraged.

Unfortunately, the HIV virus is spreading through mid-Africa without respect to the circumcision status of its males.

Circumcision status in South Africa is an interesting kaleidoscope. Whites of British ancestry are generally circumcised at birth while those of Dutch (Boer) lineage remain uncircumcised. The huge nontribal black population and the mixed "coloreds" are mostly uncircumcised, while those remaining in tribal situations still lose their foreskin to puberty-age rites.

An interesting news story from the *Johannesburg Star* of June 18, 1986, reveals tribal circumcision attitudes similar to those found in Kenya:

> An estimated 30,000 men and boys in Venda are undergoing circumcision rituals, many against their will, and scores have gone into hiding for fear of being abducted. The abductions have allegedly been authorized by the president of Venda, Chief Patrick Mphephu, in his capacity as traditional chief of the Dzanani district. Villagers claimed the Chief wanted no uncircumcised males in his state. Several teachers and pupils who had not been circumcised according to Venda custom failed to report to schools when they reopened last week. Sources confirmed that schoolteacher Mr. Willie Mukwevho was at the circumcision school and that a pupil of the Mphephu High School, Mashudu Singo, had escaped. Mashudu was abducted on Sunday from a football match. He tried to escape in a taxi, but his abductors stopped it and took him. One man, who was released from the initiation [circumcision] school, refused to talk to [reporters] about his experience for fear of reprisals.

Dear Bud,

I am 88 years old and recently I went to have my regular physical checkup. My own doctor was on vacation so a new doctor looked me over. Do you know what the young whippersnapper had the gall to say to me? "Too bad you never got circumcised," he said. Hell, the chap must have a kink about circumcision.

I have been married for 55 years, have four healthy children and nine grandchildren. Before I got married I had a girl in every port and a few boys as well. Never in all my years have I had the slightest problem being uncircumcised. I never had VD or any other kind of infection.

Grandfather

Dear Grandfather,

Of course, most uncircumcised men never have problems with their foreskin, or anything attributed to its presence. There are things that can go wrong, obviously. As Marilyn Milos of NO CIRC says, "If you have a body part, something can happen to it." An amputated earlobe isn't going to get sore. I think, Grandfather, the young doctor whippersnapper's kink might be his ego — he's got a nice cut prick so why shouldn't you have one just like his?

Dear Bud,

I am uncircumcised and recently became a diabetic. While I was in the hospital I spent considerable time remembering a statement from somewhere, "Some men prefer circumcision as a solution." I don't know where that statement came from or when I read it. What I am referring to is the fact that a circular band of my foreskin contracted while I was in the hospital as a result of my first diabetic coma. Is circumcision the only therapy for my condition?

Uncircumcised

Dear Uncircumcised,

I passed your question over to my urologist correspondent, who answers:

Your description is not unknown and, in fact, not unusual among diabetics. It has the frightening medical name of balanitis xerotica obliterans. As you can tell from the third word, the end of the process is obliteration of the pliability of the foreskin. Unfortunately, it is usually progressive and circumcision is the ultimate event.

If you have caught it as soon as the contracted circular band became evident you may be able to forestall such progression if: (1) Your diabetes is well controlled, (2) you have a loose foreskin to begin with, (3) you make every effort to be scrupulously clean, and (4) you make daily use of your fingers (up to four of them) to stretch the tight ring and use Vaseline if necessary (soapy water in a hot tub will also work, as the heat helps to loosen the skin).

Uncircumcised, be sure to tell your doctor of your desire to keep your foreskin if possible, and about your progress with the above therapy. And the best of luck, my friend.

•◊ ◊•

Dear Bud,

Blue balls is the biggest problem in my life. If I don't get a load off, my damned nuts ache for days. If I only get a partial shoot, my balls make me miserable. A doctor told me I was coming too quick and should get myself circumcised so I could pump on it longer and work up a stronger orgasm. Hell, I don't want to lose my skin. My dick is a beauty; it stretches out to a fat 8 inches and has a wide, floppy foreskin which is so loose it just hangs there like a rag. My friends dig my big wad of skin, but if the doc is right about this I might go for a clip job. What about other uncut guys? Do they suffer from sour balls?

Blue Balls

Dear Blue Balls,

Premature ejaculation happens to everyone once in a while. Just when you think you're about to explode, you only get a puny pop ... and aching balls the next day. According to my urologist: "Cut and uncut guys both have the same reasons for getting blue balls and circumcision does not affect the situation at all." A quick orgasm rarely has anything to do with your cock, he adds. It's all in your head. Think about something besides your beautiful 8 inches and its fat wad of skin. Leave that to your partner. Forget about your pending orgasm; forget how good that foreskin feels as it rolls up and down your quivering shaft.

Think about a fantasy in which sex just goes on and on and orgasm isn't being considered yet. Imagine that you are at the Roman baths. When your real orgasm explodes, let it come as a surprise to you, spontaneously. Instead of blue balls you'll have hot nuts and be ready for another session at the Roman baths — fat wad of foreskin intact. That will keep your friends happy.

●◇ ◇●

Dear Bud,

My foreskin is long and loose, but it doesn't stretch back over the shaft as far as other foreskins I've seen. If I try to stretch it back "all the way" it bends downward, as if I had a dowsing rod between my legs. People have told me I have a short frenulum. Can anything be done about a short frenulum (short of circumcision, which I don't want)?

Dowsing Rod

Dear Dowsing Rod,

Back to my urologist correspondent we go:

When the penis bends downward this is called *chordee*, usually associated with other conditions. Your condition is clearly caused by a short frenulum (frenum) and is correctable by a *frenoplasty*, rarely done except by urologists. Talk with a urologist about this. You'll be happier if you get your condition fixed. The procedure can be done under local anesthesia if your local doctor likes sticking needles into cocks. Personally, I think all penile surgery is best done under general anesthesia since swelling occurs with local injections and may not lead to the best-looking result. The operation should not put you out of commission for more than ten days, even with the stretching of a few unwanted erections.

Dowsing Rod, allow me to add that a frenoplasty need not include your circumcision. The procedure merely removes the frenulum. I received a letter from a man whose New England military school had a policy of removing the frenulum (instead of the foreskin) from each cadet. The result was long, loose foreskin on my correspondent. Tight frenulum problems, as well as crooked cocks, have also been reported by many USA members who were circumcised at birth. As my urologist suggested, however, there are many causes of "bent cocks." Only your doctor can diagnose your specific situation.

Dear Bud,

I have a penis with a bulbous glans and I am uncut. When I get rock-hard the glans just flares out in all directions and sometimes it's too much for my foreskin. My foreskin develops tiny splits right on top during sex. It doesn't hurt much but it bleeds and inevitably stops the session fast. It heals up after a few days of sexual abstinence and I've never seen a doctor about the condition because I know damn well he would recommend circumcision. Please ask your urologist friend how I can help my foreskin accommodate my fat cockhead?

Fat Cockhead

Dear Fat Cockhead,
    Okay. Doc?

These recurring tiny splits will eventually lead to scar tissue, though imperceptible, no matter how you slice it. This situation again would be ideal for foreskin stretching. I suspect that with your prow-shaped glans and its generous proportions, there may be other things that "split" besides your foreskin.

So once again, we hear that stretching is a most important (and still pleasurable) therapy for a healthy foreskin. With thumbs and fingers prodding inside the skin and pulling outward off the head, let's go ... all together now!

Dear Bud,

My pubic hairs creep inside my foreskin and it drives me crazy. My foreskin is a half-mast job that only covers half my cockhead. Whether I wear boxers, jockeys, or go naked, the hairs keep getting trapped inside my skin roll and it irritates my sensitive cockhead. If I start getting a boner in my pants it pulls at the root of my pubic hair and hurts like hell! The only way I can get the hair out of my cock is to pull my cock out of my pants, retract my foreskin, and pick each hair off one at a time. It takes time, so I can't do it at work. I just have to suffer.

I have shaved my pubes but then it itches when the hair grows back and people complain about the stiff bristles in their face. I don't want my partners to go away unhappy. Would you? Now I am considering permanent removal of my pubic hair. Could I do it myself with tweezers? Or do I have to go to a professional?

Sore Pubes

Dear Pubes,

Hair under the foreskin, as any uncircumcised man knows, is damned uncomfortable. It seldom occurs when the foreskin is long and comes to a closed, puckered tip, unless its owner neglects to pull the skin back over the head after pissing. "Half-masters" (short foreskins) seem more prone to the problem. I consulted our urologist about your complaint and he suggested, again, foreskin stretching. The problem will diminish with longer foreskin. He also suggested, "Twist your penis as you roll the foreskin forward and you'll make it almost impossible for hairs to get into the curves and crevices."

Eliminating pubic hair is not a new human practice. The Arabs have made it a mandatory ritual to cleanliness. For centuries, they have picked off one pube at a time. Having pubes is almost as sexually offensive to an Arab as having a foreskin. Of course, using tweezers is a full-time endeavor, something you could do each night before going to sleep. Check out a professional hair remover if you are really serious about being bald down there, but then you might get other complaints: "What happened to your fuckin' hair, man?"

"Pubic hair," my urologist correspondent writes, "has a texture different from other body hair and, when freshly washed, has a wonderful aroma that helps to make the sexual experience better." My advice, pal, is to think long (long foreskin), not short (short pubes), and make everybody happy.

●◇ ◇●

Dear Bud,

As a physician, I have thought more about foreskin replacement since reading the USA newsletter, and you are doing a tremendous service to bring the subject into the open. I am also interested in your observations of foreskin stretching. I have used tongs in my office practice, telling patients to stretch, but with no definite method to follow (this in cases of post-inflammatory scarring and phimosis). I never refer a case of phimosis for circumcision. Yet even as a doctor, I was unaware until recently how much of the penile "sensuality" is in the foreskin.

I don't believe smegma is detrimental in any way. I have never — I repeat, never — seen any penile condition that could be contributed to smegma. Many irritations are due to excessive cleansing (especially with certain soaps). I have four sons and in early childhood we never practiced foreskin retraction. One last item: I have a study about the effect of circumcision on the urethral meatus which indicates that the meatal calibre (the degree of urethral opening) diminishes with age in 60 percent of neonatally circumcised men. Obviously, an unnecessary operation that causes such a dramatic change in a vital orifice should be explained to the public — and it has not been! This is a gross, incredibly deliberate deception of the American public.

Physician

Dear Physician,

Thanks for your opinions and support. Yes, while we talk of all the little things that can go wrong with foreskin, we tend to overlook the potential problems of the circumcised penis. Your comment about the diminishing meatal calibre on the dried, hardening glans penis of older circumcised men is a good example. Meatal stenosis in older men usually is treated by surgery to widen the opening. One urologist wrote that his two most frequent surgical procedures are circumcising infants and performing meatotomony on circumcised adults.

Another problem with circumcision is that too much skin can be removed, causing the shaft to become so taut during erection that it causes pain. Such a condition is not uncommon among American men. One former U.S. Army medic admitted that, while stationed in Korea, he circumcised a man whose penis was too large for the surgical tool the doctor had been provided. He circumcised the man anyway and took off too much skin. The man, whose penis was far beyond average length, was sent to a plastic surgeon in Tokyo. "It was a shame," wrote the urologist, "because the man's foreskin was long and loose. We circumcised him just because he was a 'catch' — he had the biggest dick in Korea."

●◇ ◇●

Dear Bud,

I am a doctor who does not believe that circumcision is necessary. It's still a mystery to me how the anti-masturbation canard was put forward for such a long time. I recall a remark from a student in Rumania around 1939 who wrote, "Why do they want a foreskin if it isn't to help them masturbate?" I also have a difficult time understanding why so many uncircumcised doctors insist on circumcision. I know of a U.S. Navy doctor who boasted of circumcising over 6,000 sailors, but he himself was uncut. Currently I know of a British doctor, active in the Boy Scouts, giving sex talks to high-school-age boys, who claims to be very pro-circumcision, apparently loves to circumcise, and drums up business among the boys. But again, he himself is uncut.

On the other hand, the recent violent reaction against routine circumcision in Britain (beginning in 1949 and now spreading to New Zealand, Australia, and to a much lesser degree, the U.S.) is in most part advanced by doctors who are circumcised. There is no question that in 1949 the most circumcised section of British society was the medical profession. The spate of anti-circumcision articles appearing in Australia must in large part be written by circumcised doctors. There may well be exceptions, but in my experience when a circumcised man is very pro, most likely he was "done" as an adult.

Doc

Dear Doc,

Thanks for your shrewd observations. Adult circumcision, with all the subsequent changes in erotic sensation that it may involve, seems most erotic to men who can experience such a change ... to men who, at least during a part of their lives, have possessed a foreskin. What can a neonatally circumcised man know of such erotic changes? My experience with USA members is that most of our neonatally circumcised members hate the idea of circumcision and could not understand how it could possibly be erotic. The uncut members, however, whether or not they had an interest in their own circumcision, often do find the subject erotic. Most of our pro-circumcision members were, indeed, circumcised as adults or youths (at their request). I suppose it is a matter of the erotic options one has with his own penis. As I noted earlier in this book, just reading the word *circumcision* produces an erection in many uncircumcised men.

To answer your query about the anti-masturbation canard, let's review the following experience by one USA member:

I am a married father of an uncircumcised boy. I read one of your articles and was astonished to learn that surgical foreskin reconstruction was available in this country. Regaining my lost foreskin has long been a dream of mine. I have discussed it with several doctors who couldn't offer me any help but to say it was all in my mind. They didn't know how I felt — or feel — about myself.

I was circumcised under rather bizarre circumstances and have always resented my circumcision. I want to share my story with your readers in hopes that another boy can be spared a similar experience. My problem began just after my sixteenth birthday when my parents galloped off to Europe and left my brother and me in the charge of our grandmother (whom we really didn't like), a very old-fashioned lady who was inclined to snoop. One day I was in the bathroom masturbating when the door slightly opened and there she was. At first I thought that because of her failing eyesight she hadn't realized what was going on. But she had.

Up to that time my foreskin completely covered the glans. It hung down about $1/2$" over the end of my penis and was loose, with no rosette. My father was also uncircumcised, as is my brother. I never had any problems with my foreskin, as it retracted completely and was easy to keep clean.

Three days after the incident in the bathroom, I was told "we" were going to the doctor and off we went, with me not knowing what for, other than she probably wanted an escort as she was seeing him for one of her problems. When we arrived I was ushered into a room, then was told to strip and put on the gown that hung on the door. Very shortly I was taken into another room and told to lay on the table. I was strapped across the chest, arms, as well as my legs. Next the nurse folded the gown up, exposing me, and started to shave me. It was the first time a woman had seen me and my penis was as erect as it had ever been. It was extremely embarrassing. She continued on, handling me to the bitter end. Then came a wash with some smelly stuff and a towel was put over me. By now I had an idea what was in store for me but with the restraints there was nothing I could do.

Soon the doctor came in and the fun started. I begged and pleaded to a pair of deaf ears — absolutely no response on his part — as he washed and put on the surgical gloves. The nurse switched on the lights above the table and he pulled my penis out through a hole in the towel, pulled my foreskin as far forward as it would go, and administered two shots of anesthetic. By now it was hard again despite the needle and he had to wait a minute or two. He put in three more shots, skinned it back, and put another shot in the frenulum. He laid an open pair of blunt scissors on the glans, drew my foreskin up over this instrument, and made a cut right over the center of the glans.

At this point I was dumbfounded, hurt, humiliated — you name it. I couldn't watch anymore. Finally he said he was finished, and the gown was pulled back down. They had me sit on the table for a while and then told me to get dressed. Naturally, when the gown was off I looked down and was amazed to see the black threads (sutures) holding gauze squares around my glans. I dressed and was told to return in five days and headed home alone (my grandmother had long since departed). On the way home the anesthetic began to wear off and a burning sensation started which became worse and worse and lasted about three days before it let up. I was plagued with erections constantly, which were very painful as they pulled on the stitches. The visit on the fifth day was to remove the stitches. As a parting shot the doctor said to me, "Now you won't play with yourself anymore." Boy, was he wrong!

The immediate reaction was extreme sensitivity of the glans. There was no pain, but the slightest friction from my clothing gave me a raging hard-on. Shortly after school was to open, my parents returned and that evening I showed my father what had happened. He was furious. He had a big, loud fight with my grandmother (my mother's mother) and the family rift lasted until her dying day. In school there were about thirty-five boys in the gym showers and as I recall, about twelve of us had been uncircumcised. It never seemed to make much difference although the circumcised boys often stared at those of us with foreskins. Now it was an entirely different story. My glans was still a deep pink and the scars were red and ugly — nobody could miss it. I got a razzing from cut and uncut boys alike. As a direct result, I became very self-conscious of my penis, which I had never been before, and felt barer than bare in the presence of other nude men. I still feel as if I am permanently naked.

Still Sore

Dear Bud,

I was eleven years old when my father died. My mother hated him and his "filthy" uncut dick. It had been his demand that my brother and I not be circumcised when we were born. After his death, the first thing she did was send us to a medical school to get circumcised. She couldn't afford to send us to a private doctor. I was terrified. As a result, I have a lifelong distrust of doctors ever since and I hate my mother.

My penis still had huge red scars when I returned to school and one day while I was at a urinal two boys surrounded me. One of them ran a knife around my cock and said tauntingly, "We know what they did to you. We know what they did to you." Do you wonder why I have joined the anti-circumcision campaign?

Lifetime Member

Dear Anti-Circumcision People,

Insensitivity toward a boy's penis seems to have been prevalent until recently. I recall the famous quote from a turn-of-the-century English doctor when asked if he enjoyed his profession: "My only regret is that I am called upon to gaze at nature's most hideous creation, the male genitals."

No wonder they didn't mind chopping off English foreskins in his day! Today, most physicians have a very different attitude. As a urologist wrote to the USA, "We must not forget that the penis is a cosmetic organ. It is man's avenue towards social and marital happiness."

The USA received many letters from men circumcised in their postinfancy boyhood. Their resulting trauma has led most of them to be avid anti-circumcisionists. To again quote Dr. Spock's article in *Redbook:*

> Boys, especially between the ages of two and four, tend to become quite anxious about the safety of their penises. It is at this time that they usually become aware that little girls don't have a penis ... When an older boy is circumcised, even though the body of the penis remains, the circumcision suggests to the child that an attempt has been made to cut the penis off and, in fact, the attempt has been partially successful.

Dear Bud,

I got myself circumcised at nineteen because I had always fantasized about my father's circumcised penis. He was circumcised as a boy and hated it, that's why he wouldn't allow his sons to get clipped. He might have hated his dick, but I spent my boyhood dreaming about owning a handsomely circumcised penis just like his.

Dad's Boy

Dear Boy,

You might have a handsomely circumcised penis now, but there is one big difference between you and your father; circumcision was your choice, while I doubt that your father had that choice. To be able to choose one's own penis style is, indeed, fortunate.

Dear Bud,

I dig the looks of the big, tough-headed, sleek all-American clipcock. I prefer the "back to the balls" variety which have the frenulum area trimmed smooth and a prominent circumcision ring about halfway up the pole. Most of the guys I grew up with had my idolized dick swinging between their legs and I always felt left out. I've always wanted to be circumcised but I think I waited too long. I am in my early thirties and I understand that when an adult gets circumcised he ends up with stitch marks instead of a manly looking scar and they usually leave a lot of loose skin on the penis because of the huge difference in size between flaccid and erect. I know that many adult-circumcised men have written to you. What are your observations about their restyled dicks?

Left Out

Dear Left Out,

It's never too late to get circumcised, nor to get a "back to the balls" tight job. I am not promoting adult circumcision except in the context that it might be preferable to infant circumcision. You, my friend, still have a choice. All those fellows you grew up with probably didn't choose to have that all-American clipcock swinging between their legs. True, I receive many letters from adult-circumcised men, but I have received even more from men circumcised at birth who resent not having had that choice. So, Left Out, the choice is still before you. Enjoy the possibilities.

Yes, most adult-circumcised penises do have stitches ringing their shafts, and they are not sleekly skinned. I've received many letters from men dissatisfied with their adult circumcisions for that very reason, many of whom have gone back for a second and even third circumcision to get the "back-to-the balls" look they want. I personally know one young man who chose to be circumcised at fifteen (the only uncut boy in his one-room school) and again at eighteen, and his shaft is "sleek." Most doctors, however, are apprehensive about cutting off too much skin. I've heard horror stories which ended with a man going to a plastic surgeon because his tight skin ached.

Stitches can be a problem, but while the young man mentioned above has such stitches, they're almost imperceptible. Remember, Left Out, that circumcision is surgery and all surgery involves risks. There is also the psychological effect of adapting to a newly styled penis. I had a letter from a priest whose reaction to adult circumcision was so negative that he had to wear cotton over his bared glans for several years. Others are able to start sexual activity within weeks, and are delighted with the results. Two factors seem especially important in determining one's reaction to adult circumcision: the condition of the foreskin before it was cut off, and whether the desire for the circumcision was erotic.

Men with tight foreskins and supersensitive, extremely moist glans should consider circumcision warily because the change could be very radical. Men with long, loose foreskins whose glans are relatively dry are more easily circumcised — there's lots of inner foreskin with which to work — and they adopt to the change more easily. Men with short foreskin, according to my correspondents, hardly notice any before-and-after difference in their penises, making one wonder why they bothered.

Reasons for the adult circumcision are important. Medical reasons, of course, are one thing, and I don't intend to question them here. Social reasons, such as "everybody else has an all-American clipcock" or "my lover prefers a circumcised cock," can lead to great disappointment. Eroticism should be a factor in the desire for an adult circumcision. After all, a man's entire erotic life is on the chopping block.

The Acorn Club (the support group for pre- and postcircumcised adult men) requires that their candidates prove desire for circumcision by an erection. Acorn membership is mostly heterosexual men who have a lifetime fixation on circumcision. You might consider their interest to be the result of their American childhood with "different" uncircumcised penises. However, there's an Acorn Club in uncircumcised England too, and both clubs have members in Europe as well as in Asia. A test the Acorns used to determine acceptance of a member is placing him naked before a full-length mirror and making him repeat over and over, "circumcision, circumcision." If his chant gives him an erection, then he's a candidate. He's made the choice!

●◆ ◆●

Dear Buddy Bud,

I feel I can tell you my secret. I want to get circumcised. I dig having foreskin and I have no medical problems with it, but the thought of having it cut off drives me wild. Every time I see the word "circumcision" in print I get a hard-on. Every time I re-read your articles, I read with a stiff pole between my legs. I met this big dude and he turned on to my skin something fierce. He tied me down and shouted things like "I hate skinheads!" and "filthy punk." Then he stretched my skin out wide and hot-waxed it, and proceeded to clamp it with clothespins. Then he really turned mean and shouted, "I'm going to rip that goddamn skin off your dick!" My poor cock was sore but rock-hard when I shouted, "Rip it off! Rip it off!" The bastard was too chicken to circumcise me. How do I join Acorn? I've got an erection to show them.

●◇ ◇●

Dear Bud,

My girlfriend and I are swingers. We share a fantasy about finding a handsome uncircumcised man for a three-some, tying him down, and circumcising him without his permission. Do you have any candidates in the USA?

●◇ ◇●

Dear Bud,

I am a Marine in San Diego and am one of the few around who's still got his roll, as far as I've seen. Once in a while I get a craving for real hot action on my skin. I dig having it pulled, stretched, licked, chewed, hot-waxed, stuck with pins, sewn shut. Anything goes, as long as my sex-skin gets all the attention, I don't give a shit if I get blown or even come ... just skin action!

The only ones I've found who know how to handle my hot skin are a couple of older dudes in Frisco, and when my roll starts telling me, "Hey, man, don't forget me down here!" I hop on my Harley and spend a weekend with those old bruisers while they make me glad as hell I've still got my skin.

●◇ ◇●

Dear Bud,

I was circumcised at a Texas prison farm as punishment for an attempted escape. Now my younger brother wants to have his beautiful long foreskin cut off, too. I'm trying to talk him out of it because he hasn't done anything wrong to be circumcised for.

●◇ ◇●

Dear Bud,

I recall a bunch of my college buddies heading into Mexico for spring break. We were driving through a remote, rural area when the cops pulled us over. We were taken to a rinky-dink police office and strip-searched for drugs. They didn't find any until one officer pointed to the dick of the only uncut guy in the bunch. Sure enough, he had pot hidden up his foreskin. We all watched while a so-called doctor cut off his foreskin without painkiller. Afterwards, we were told we could go free because, "No place to hide it next time." I still think they planted the stuff up my buddy's skin just to have some fun with us.

Dear Circumcising People,

Circumcision has often been used as a punishment. Back in 1977 I read a story in the *Chicago Tribune* about a trial in the South. A prisoner admitted that he had confessed to a crime, but said it was only after a police officer threatened to circumcise him.

Why is the act of circumcision also an act of sadism? Why have we had thousands of years of sadism directed at that small part of human anatomy? Why is it erotic to cut off the foreskin of some pubertal boy, an unsuspecting "handsome man," or a prisoner? Why is an uncircumcised man willing to stand in front of a mirror, staring at his erection, chanting, "circumcision, circumcision"?

B.Z. Goldberg, in his classic book *The Sacred Fire*, gives some insight on this issue. Referring to the one sado-masochistic human experience institutionalized by heterosexuals — the moment at which the bridegroom must break the hymen, which symbolically represents the transition from virginity to the realm of sexual experience — Goldberg writes:

> The foreskin is the nearest to [the female hymen]. Like the hymen, it undergoes a change in sexual intercourse. Again,

like the hymen, it can be removed with pain, yet with little danger to the life of the individual. We thus have circumcision at the time of puberty as a sacrifice of the male agent in the sexual process.

Or, in the words of the military medic I quoted previously: "What are you complaining about? I've made a man out of you!"

●◇ ◇●

Dear Bud,
I think you have been too harsh on the Arabs as the perpetrators of circumcision. You seem to stereotype them all as sword-swinging fanatics. Certainly they have changed their attitudes about the forced circumcision of prisoners since the days of the Crusades. If any people are fanatic about circumcision it is the Jews, and I think they are the major cause of American circumcision.
Pinpointing the
True Perpetrator

Dear Perpetrator,
True, my history has been harsh on the Moslems. Keep in mind, however, that not all Moslems are Arabs, nor are all Arabs Moslems. Historically, the Sword of Islam did play the major role in the British lineage of American routine circumcision, although the sword was swung most effectively by the non-Arabic Moguls of India. The Arabs of High Islam contributed immensely to a Europe just awakening from the Dark Ages: They contributed fine art and architecture, tile, printed fabric, the clean-shaven face for the male ... and also for the male, the concept of the circumcised penis. Many of these contributions entered Europe with returning Crusaders — knights who, in some cases, had joined secret societies emulating the occult initiation rites of the Fatimid rulers of Egypt. One such rite was circumcision.

The Jews also contributed to European culture but, as far as religious practice is concerned, we can make one major distinction between the two Semitic religions: Modern Judaism is not prone to proselytism while Islam is aggressive about it. The Jews have rarely urged religious circumcision on other populations, while the Sword of Islam has turned entire male populations into "Believers." In recent history, Islam has had little influence on Western culture, while the Jews have had a profound influence. It would be easy to point the finger at Jewish doctors, accusing them of promoting circumcision. Of course, many Jewish doctors have promoted clinical circumcision, but no more than many Gentile doctors. I know of several Jewish doctors who are influential in today's anti-circumcision movement. Jewish clergymen certainly don't promote the circumcision of Gentiles, preferring to keep their "covenant" sacred to themselves.

Is the Sword of Islam still swinging at foreskins as it was during the time of the Crusades? Let me quote from the experience of a USA member who was an American consul to Indonesia during the 1960s:

> I was invited to attend a combined family celebration in the village where my night watchman in Jakarta came from. His sister was fourteen and his brother was seven. The sister was marrying a boy of sixteen and the brother was getting circumcised. As the afternoon festivities proceeded the boy was circumcised on the front lawn with a multitude of onlookers. Afterwards, the circumciser and myself as honored guests were seated next to each other for the feast. Being uncircumcised, I felt very uneasy sitting next to a real live circumciser.
>
> I could think of nothing else but circumcision around which to make small talk with him. I mentioned that I had read about Moslems in Mogul India circumcising English prisoners. The circumciser smiled and said, "I guess you think that kind of practice ended a long time ago? Well, not so! I myself have forcibly circumcised POWs during our war of independence from the Dutch (1945–49)." At this announcement I felt my penis begin to swell and my masochistic eroticism came to the fore. He explained that the Indonesian Christians supported the Dutch rule and joined the KNIL (Royal Dutch Indies army). When they were captured they were taken back to a patriot (Moslem) village and forced to strip naked before they were publicly circumcised one by one. He added, "They did not use anesthetic, like had been used on the boy I just circumcised in the garden, but

carved the male organs with the benefit of full sensation."

With my heart pounding and my penis straining, I gingerly asked, "Did you circumcise every prisoner of war?"

"Absolutely, every male prisoner was circumcised," was his quick reply. "I mean," I nervously asked, "Did you circumcise Dutchmen too?" He laughed and said, "Of course." I excused myself from the dinner table...

While I was stationed in Indonesia I became aware of a troublesome Moslem group on the Island of Sulawesi (Celebes) called Dural Islam. They tried to overthrow Sukarno's government since he had not made Indonesia an official Moslem state. A friend told me the following stories of the warfare that ensued: "The Darul Islam had burned bare an entire area and took between 500 and 700 males of all ages to the forest with them. All the prisoners, including Torajad, Chinese, and Europeans, were forcibly circumcised. In South Salawesi, they were particularly cruel against the POWs of the Indonesian army sent against them. They cut off their penises, which were then tied to trees to show how many of the enemy had fallen to their arms."

Perpetrator, why do I get a sense of *déjà vu?* Isn't this where we started our history of the foreskin? Foreskins and penises being whacked off in Biblical times? Some things change, but the penis and its foreskin remain a target. I certainly don't intend to indict the Muslim religion for the actions of a few fanatics. In the case of circumcision, however, I believe that religion has sanctified an erotic urge. After all, it was our American consul whose uncircumcised penis stood at attention upon hearing of the Moslem forced circumcisions. If you ask me, the principal designers of the great all-American clipcock were not the Jews or the Moslems, but our own fanatical Protestant-puritanical anti-masturbationists.

NOTES

1. U.P.I. news story, Dec. 6, 1986.

2. Adrian MacFarlane, "What a Baby Knows," *Human Nature,* Feb. 1978, p. 74.

3. Aaron Fink, M.D., in "To Circumcise or Not to Circumcise?" *Stanford Medicine*, Spring 1988, p. 17.

4. These were reported by Harold V. Kunz, M.D., in his article "Circumcision and Meatotomy," in *Primary Care*, Sept. 1986, p. 513.

3. Icons, Numbers, Choices

Dear Bud,

I really dig the look of an uncircumcised penis when the foreskin is fully forward in a natural position, but it makes me curious about what is hidden inside. I suppose my imagination goes to work when I can't see the whole works.

Dig Secrets

Dear Dig,

Okay, just for you we'll scat back.

Dear Bud,

Can you verify that the King of Rock and Roll was uncircumcised? I am a devoted fan of Elvis Presley and would be overjoyed to learn that such a beautiful man was uncircumcised.

Elvis Fan

Dear Fan,

Yes, the King was uncircumcised. Several years ago, Albert Goldman's biography *Elvis* set off a wave of controversy about his penis. I received the following letter from the editor of *Elvis World* magazine:

Dear Mr. Berkeley,

Your organization has been recommended to us by one of your readers in hopes you can offer a statement regarding the degrading remarks made by the author, Albert Goldman, in his best-selling biography, a very degrading account of the life of the King, himself uncircumcised.

Mr. Goldman writes that Elvis "saw his beauty disfigured by an ugly hillbilly pecker." Not only is this generalization in bad taste, but it is not verifiable. Mr. Berkeley, would you comment on Mr. Goldman's statement for us, please?

I replied in an article published in *Drummer* magazine:

In the fifties, the only time foreskin was mentioned was in jest. Chances are what Mr. Goldman is referring to was a remark Elvis made humorously. Certainly if being uncircumcised bothered Elvis, he had the money to get circumcised. The very fact that he was in the Army and got out with foreskin intact suggests that he must have been pretty firm about keeping it."

That Presley was uncircumcised was verified by the wide publication of his death certificate, which had a check after the designation "uncircumcised." Some states make such a designation as an aid to identification. Speculation about whether Elvis really disliked being uncut was complicated by author Goldman's convincing argument that the only reason he didn't get circumcised was his great fear of "the knife." It was certainly true that when the King was waving his hips at audiences, the penis he was pushing in his pants was very unfashionable. He wasn't the only uncircumcised American who felt disfigured. Hey, King, times have changed.

●◇ ◇●

Dear Bud,

I attended college in France and realized immediately that I was at home there. I can't tell you the relief it was to be among other uncircumcised men. I spent my vacations at the nudist *Ile du Levant*. Almost all the males on the beach were uncut and I enjoyed watching those lovely cocks with their great variety of foreskins. I was fascinated. Some men with small cocks had long foreskins and some men had just enough foreskin so that the pisshole barely peeked through. I watched one young blond guy play volleyball for hours. His lovely, pointed foreskin kept slipping back and forth so naturally that he couldn't keep his penis from throbbing when his team was being victorious.

Love Watching Lovely Cocks

Dear Watching,

Ah, yes! The French have such pretty penises. Unlike some of the Germanic groups in Europe, the French prefer their men to have small, thin penises with long, tapered foreskins, Hellenistic-style — not that all French penises are small by any means, but they don't generally worry about cock size. The Germans, on the other hand, prefer voluptuous, fat penises with wide, floppy foreskin that retracts easily, Roman-style — not that all German penises are large. But Europe is so full of foreskin, of all varieties and types, that at any time on the nude beaches of southern France or northern Germany an American can receive an education just by using a pair of binoculars.

Overall, Europe has a circumcision rate of 10 percent, mostly the result of diagnosed phimosis. Most penises with the "European Cut"–style circumcision have an amazing amount of skin remaining on the shaft, sometimes many folds of it. Also amazing is that all the loose shaft skin never touches the glans or its corona. And, as most European circumcisions take place during youth, rather than at birth, their glans are smooth, sensitive, and undamaged.

The fact that the French and Germans are 90 percent uncircumcised today is really a fluke of history when you consider the English and Americans. Recall that both nations considered universal circumcision during the nineteenth century as a prevention of masturbation. "Pretty penises," as it turned out, were more important to the French than circumcision. However, the military classes of both France and Germany, just as in Britain, went through a period of "bearing the mark."

The Manly Arts catalog that I've already mentioned offered delicious tidbits of circumcision history, including some that reflects the French and German experience. The catalog offered for sale (asking price $5000) an original

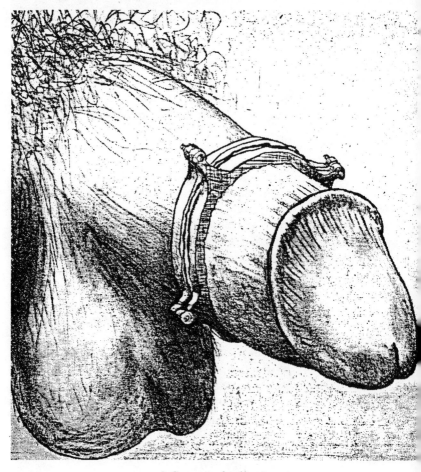

A German **bediente**

French "Gasconade Kit" with the following description:

> "The French origin of this item should not be overlooked.
> Louis XVI was the first French monarch to be circumcised.
> The young nobility soon emulated him. After the revolution,
> circumcision was adopted by the Incroyables ['Those who
> dress incredibly']. The Incroyables were the hippies of their
> day. 'Gasconade' means a person who boasts or brags."

While the Incroyables might have bragged about their
circumcised cocks, they must have been pretty brave to
survive the Gasconade Kit. The Manly Arts catalogue described the machine: "Operated by seizing the foreskin with

nibbled rings, sending a plunger down into the foreskin to push the glans out of danger and then, by a turn of the crank, sending a blade through the foreskin."

The Germans were represented in the Manly Arts catalogue by *bediente*, or retainer, circa 1910. Similar in purpose to the anti-circumcision rings being sold in America, the *bediente* attempted to avoid circumcision by permanently retracting the foreskin. According to Manly Arts: "One must assume that the foreskin was folded internally and the bediente used to keep it in place. One must also ask about the clumsiness of such a device, its difficulty in being placed, the curious outlines it must have created, and the sensations experienced by one's partners."

Modern Germans have not completely escaped the knife. During the days of Communist domination of East Germany, the chief medical officer of the East German police, a Dr. Diatz, pushed through an ordinance ordering the circumcision of all male police personnel. He designed his own circumcision tool, made of bone, which crushed the doomed foreskin at the place of excision. Reportedly he, himself, performed the honors during the initial years of the ordinance and did so with great gusto. He had an entire corps of foreskins to crush. I supposed, upon first hearing of Diatz's fun and games, that he was a sadist or, possibly, that his motive was to have the only circumcised penises in Europe as a mark of "identification" for East German spies. However, as a result of his ordinance, neonatal circumcision of East German infants enjoyed a brief popularity.

•◇ ◇•

Dear Bud,

An extraordinary thing happened at my gymnasium the other night. While sitting in the steam room I found myself alone with three other uncircumcised fellows. That is as many as I've seen in the entire place in one night. Of course, I felt like speaking out but I didn't know any of these guys. One of them caught me studying his cock. He smiled and repaid the compliment. We both glanced around at the other cocks in the room and our eyes returned to meet with the most surprised look! We started to laugh quietly. The other two men looked up wondering what was so funny. They soon caught on and there we sat, four rare birds ... young, uncircumcised Americans ... alone in a big-city steam room. Nothing was said. Gradually, all four dicks began to rise.

Then slowly, hesitantly, we each began to masturbate — we didn't know which fellow was gay or straight. It didn't matter as our strokes got more intense. We were watching each other pump our foreskins, curious about techniques. Long, slow motions with a tight fist right over the cockhead ... steady beat. We all had the exact same stroke. One fellow stopped stroking and pulled his foreskin back off his glans, I suppose to demonstrate his retraction ability. We all followed his lead. All loose. We kept our skins back long enough to compare our glans, which were all redder than most, softer in texture than most, each with a different shape. We released our foreskins simultaneously and watched them gradually creep up the long, stiff shaft and slowly swallow the glans, each one stopping at a different preordained location on the penis. Suddenly, the door opened and in walked the outside world ... the circumcised world.

Fourth Musketeer

Dear Bud,

I was shooting a 16mm adventure film from Suez to Mersa Alam, mostly underwater. In the south we got into more remote areas and filmed near Egyptian army outposts of Camel Corps soldiers. These men rode daily from one outpost to the next, keeping an eye out for any invasion from across the Red Sea. They soon became acquainted with our film crew and began to hang around our sets. We were swimming naked in the sea one day when the temperature was at least 116 degrees. They sat on their camels and smiled at us. I noticed they were tugging at their crotches.

On several occasions when I took my camera and swam a mile or more up the coast, I would swim ashore to reload the camera. One such time I thought I was alone on the desert shore when I looked up to find myself surrounded by three Egyptian soldiers on camelback. I was stark naked. That didn't seem to bother them as they literally led me to their tent at the top of a small sand dune. They insisted on serving me tea. As I sat with them, one reached out and touched my cock, asking why it wasn't circumcised. I explained that I came from a Christian family which didn't believe in circumcision. Anyway, they all had to touch my penis and push the foreskin back and forth. I was quite surprised by their boldness. I then learned that I was expected to return the compliment: I had to inspect each Egyptian circumcised penis. That was it. I returned to the shore for my swim back to the film set, while my hosts hollered and whooped their fond farewell. I figured that the whole episode was merely an expression of male camaraderie.

Sphinx

●◇ ◇●

Dear Bud,

I recently returned from a mission in Central Africa where I had spent three years teaching school. When I arrived there I was uncircumcised and the people with whom I worked were from a tribe that performed ritual circumcision at puberty. The men were extremely tall, elegantly proportioned, and their long, circumcised penises made me feel inferior. I was warmly welcomed into their lives; I lived naked with them and was considering their offer of allowing me to join the next group of youths to be circumcised.

However, before that was possible circumcision became a medical necessity for me, as I was bitten by a certain type of mosquito which caused elephantiasis (gross swelling of the scrotum and penis). It became so swollen that treatment was difficult and the mission doctor circumcised me under very crude conditions while eight of his African aide-in-firmers watched. After the operation they invited me to go through their ritual exercises, one of which was to face a line of men who whipped me as I ran back and forth between them naked — this little game was the fate of their boys prior to circumcision. Then, members of three tribes mixed their blood with the blood from my penis and I proudly became their blood brother. I must say I like myself circumcised because this was the way I bonded with African men.

Blood Brother

Dear Bud,

I am a football coach at a small New England college. I've never considered myself to be gay, but I have always been interested in the bodies of my athletes. I suppose it's natural for a coach to be proud of his men, both in their appearance and their performance. If I wasn't interested in the male body I probably wouldn't be a coach. I think there is nothing more magnificent than a well-toned physique. It is nature's most perfect instrument. I seldom go into the showers so I don't see my men naked very often. When I watch them on the field, I sometimes strip them in my head, fantasizing about their genitals. Frankly, I always picture their penises as being whole. Uncircumcised. I couldn't bear to think that any of those perfect human specimens has been mutilated by circumcision. Of course, I am prejudiced because I, myself, am uncut. I suppose a feeling of male camaraderie is more possible between men who have the same circumcision status.

Coach

Dear Bud,

When I started school, I had gym for the first time. When we went to the shower room, the boys were in all states of development ... but I was the only one with a foreskin. There was much staring, but nothing else.

By the next day at gym period, the kids decided to make fun of me and I got into a fight. It was stopped by the gym teacher who made me go to his office after school for reprimand as a troublemaker. When he asked why I started the fight I told him they were making fun of my prick because I wasn't circumcised. He asked if I thought there was anything wrong with not being circumcised and I told him no and that my father had told me about it.

As we talked, the most important thing he told me was that he, too, was uncircumcised. Then he explained that as I got older I would have "wet dreams" and would have to be careful to wash under my skin. I felt great knowing that the coach was like me and not like all the other guys, but I knew they wouldn't believe me if I told them he was uncircumcised.

182

The next day I expected more trouble in the gym class but when shower time came, the coach showered with us. Imagine the boys' surprise when they saw his penis. There wasn't a word, just silence. We all admired him and when they saw that he had a foreskin, mine was okay too.

Coach's Buddy

Dear Camaraderie People,

Yes, male comradeship sometimes involves the circumcision status — either out of curiosity, or maybe from ignorance and fear. As humans, we tend to fear those things we don't understand, and we shun them. As males, the one thing we do understand most intimately is our own penis. As gregarious beings we are curious about each other and tend to want others to be like ourselves. More importantly, those things different from us make us insecure, especially when our sexuality is concerned. Insecurity, in turn, often heightens erotic stresses ... and makes us curious.

Dear Bud,

When I was a young boy, my parents took me to Europe, and in Italy we saw the statue of David. I was mesmerized. It was the most beautiful piece of art I had ever seen. But I was terribly disturbed by David's cock. It sure didn't look like mine. Returning to our hotel, I quickly went to bathroom, pulled out my dick, and tried my damndest to pull skin over the top just like I had seen on the statue. I started to cry and my father came in. He explained that I had been streamlined like all American boys and that *David* was sculpted long ago and his penis was old-fashioned. To this day, whenever I see an "old-fashioned" penis on a statue, it makes me want to cry.

Memories of Italy

Dear Bud,

I was a circumcised boy who used to stare at my art book for hours, studying the photo of Michelangelo's *David*.

Davidophile

●◇ ◇●

Dear Bud,

As a student of the Bible, I just don't understand why the statue *David* has a foreskin. Surely Michelangelo knew that Jews were a circumcised race. How could he have made such a mistake?

Curious

Dear *David* People,

Like many boys, my schoolboy chum Emory and I spent hours studying the Greek and Roman statues in art books. David and his beautiful foreskin somehow gave credence to our own foreskins. After receiving many letters about *David* from USA members, I wrote the following article for one of our earlier publications (*Foreskin Quarterly* #7, copublished by Desmodus, Inc., and the USA) titled "The Most Famous Foreskin in the World":

> On January 25, 1504, the world's most famous foreskin was unveiled before the eyes of the world's most famous artists, including Leonardo da Vinci. Since his unveiling, David has been showing off his foreskin along with his magnificent male physique and well-exposed genitals for all the world to see. And the world has certainly been looking. Michelangelo's 13 $^1/_2$-foot-high statue of David has been the epitome of male beauty for almost five hundred years, and that beauty includes a foreskin. *David*, second only to the Statue of Liberty, is the world's most famous statue.
>
> David's magnificently hewed foreskin, with its deft outlining of the hidden glans and its delicately pointed overhang, is controversial. Many *David* replicas hide his most beautiful part with fig leaves, including the *David* standing so shyly in Hollywood's Forest Lawn. But the real controversy is not with David's nakedness, it is with his foreskin. As one man wrote me, "*David* is the greatest art fraud in history!" Another wrote, "Certainly Michelangelo was a learned man and a Catholic; he must have known the real David was circumcised." Another writer: "I don't understand how the artist who painted the Sistine Chapel ceiling could have made such a mistake!"
>
> The "real" David, the Prince of Judea who became King of the Jews, with a foreskin on his penis? David, who was

most certainly circumcised on his eighth day of life, and who (1 Samuel 18:27) cut off the foreskins of two hundred captured Philistines, really shouldn't be remembered as Michelangelo chiseled him ... at least not his cock. Why did the renowned artist give him a foreskin? There have been many theories bantered about: 1) The Italians of that day couldn't stand the sight of a circumcised penis; 2) Michelangelo chiseled *David* using a live model who had a foreskin; and 3) Michelangelo was not a scholar and had no idea that the Hebrews circumcised their sons.

The truth is that when the 26-year-old Michelangelo was commissioned by the Board of Works of the Cathedral of Florence, he was being asked to create a male statue called *Il Gigante*. Yes, the Florentines, who adored the finished statue which stood on a platform on the Palazzo Vecchio for all the world to see, didn't call it *David* but, instead, *The Giant*. To them, the magnificent nude male giant was a symbol of the proud, restored republic. There is no evidence that Michelangelo knew that the foreskin he chiseled out of marble would end up being considered that of David.

Michelangelo was not a theological scholar and didn't even read or understand Latin. He came from a good background for his day, but his schooling stopped at thirteen, when he was apprenticed to the artist Domenico Ghirlandaio, and his entire life thereafter was devoted to art. He loved the male physique, but unlike the flamboyant Leonardo da Vinci, whom he disliked, Michelangelo had few close relationships. He disliked women and didn't want them in his home. He was not an attractive man, even in his youth, and was often ill-tempered and, according to historian Will Durant, had only one confidante, his servant Francesco, who "for many years shared his bed."

Probably the greatest influence on the young Michelangelo as he chiseled away at the huge hunk of marble was not a lover or a model, and certainly not the original David, but those magnificent ancient Hellenist statues he studied as a student in Rome. He had just returned from Rome when he was commissioned to do *David*, and those early Greek gods were clearly in his vision, as were their foreskins. Well, call him what you will, *David* or the *The Giant*, Michelangelo created the most beautiful man in the world, complete with foreskin.

As art historian Rolf Schott wrote in his biography of the artist, *David* "radiates a nameless beauty; the pristine beauty of man in the Garden of Eden, perhaps never expressed so perfectly in the history of art."

●◇ ◇●

Dear Bud,

My husband brought your book home, and since I am the letter writer in this household, I am taking my typewriter in hand to encourage more women to write letters and experiences to you. You may underestimate your silent female audience.

I, for one, have been turned on by the sight and touch of cock as long as I can remember. My husband's foreskin is a beauty. It is long, loose, and delicate, fitting neatly over the bulging cockhead and sliding back like a sleeve until every fold vanishes. Without his foreskin, sucking would be like playing a violin with only one string. The foreskin gives me more control to hold back my husband's climax.

With suction I pull the foreskin out to its full length to tickle the tip and roll it under my tongue, before slipping my tongue between the skin and the head for some side-to-side motion. Then I press the skin halfway back to work on the head and the skin at the same time. I like to slide the smooth skin back and forth with my hand to watch the cock smile at me. Men, who were born with a penis, can't imagine how interesting a cock can be in all its changing moods. The foreskin adds to the cock's artistry.

Part of Your Female Audience

Dear Female Audience,

All I can add to your honesty is to say that your husband is a lucky man.

●◇ ◇●

Dear Bud,

I am a woman who seldom knows whether my partner is circumcised or uncircumcised. I only see their penises when they are erect and they all look alike to me. Seen

186

one and you've seen them all. And I've...

...Seen Them All

Dear Seen Them All,

Here's your study lesson for today:

Exhibit (A) is an erect uncircumcised penis and (B) is an erect circumcised penis. By the way, a lot of men out there can't tell the difference either. In fact, I've encountered both men and boys who don't know their own circumcision status.

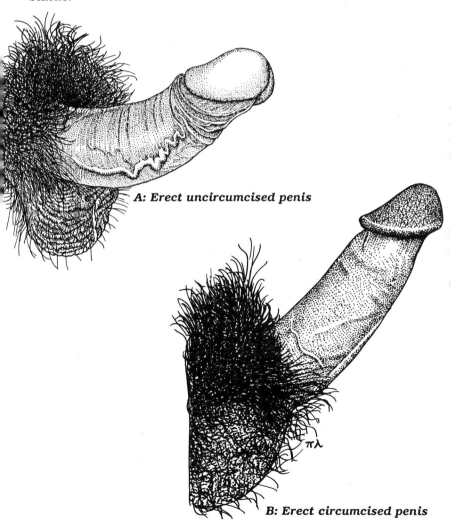

A: Erect uncircumcised penis

B: Erect circumcised penis

◆◇ ◇◆

Dear Bud,

I finally got my foreskin restoration, and none too soon. I started life with a very well done circumcision. But now that I am uncircumcised, my wife of twenty-five years is happier and we respond to each other like youngsters. She has gone through changes with age, and her vagina is often quite dry. My new slippery foreskin can be juicy enough for both of us. By the way, there is a little trick I learned in intercourse with an uncircumcised penis. If I hold her tightly when I am inside her, I can feel my cap going in and out of the foreskin. She likes the feeling of the shaft sliding in its foreskin case against her vaginal walls. When you've been married to the same woman as long as I have, a little variety is hard to come by. I can tell you that my modified tool has brought a new dimension to her interest in me.

Old Dog with New Tricks

◆◇ ◇◆

Dear Bud,

I was circumcised at fifty. It rejuvenated and changed my sex life completely. I am now much more aware of my cockhead. Before my circumcision, all my sensitivity was in my foreskin and I suppose it either dulled with age or I became bored. Now I can't wait to penetrate with my newly flaring glans and feel its raw nerves as it gives my wife new sensations.

Young Again

◆◇ ◇◆

Dear Bud,

I've been using the BUFF stretching method of foreskin restoration for the past twenty-two months. Having been tightly circumcised at birth with no excess skin, I had to use tape straps across the glans for ten months before I developed enough skin and mobility to hold the skin forward of the glans with a tape ring. After using a tape ring for the next five months, there was enough skin to require some means by which to 'extend' the skin beyond the glans in order to achieve further gain. At that point, I became very discouraged and wasn't sure I would be able to continue the stretching program.

My particular problem is that I have very tender and sensitive skin. Even hypoallergenic surgical tape irritates me unless I change its location every few days. Also, my skin is very sensitive to moisture, particularly if materials such as silicone, plastic, or rubber are involved. According to the BUFF method, if I wear objects within the foreskin which fit over, or in front of, the glans during the later stages of stretching, I must either urinate through or around them (and regularly remove them for cleaning), or remove them each time for urinating. Given the characteristics of my skin, I simply could not remove the tape repeatedly without skin damage, or urinate through an object without immediate skin reaction to the moist surface that resulted.

I experimented with various extension methods for about a month before I hit on an alternative taping method. This has allowed me not only to continue stretching but to make my most steady progress to date.

Not being a physician, I would not presume to provide medical advice in any form. I am willing, however, to describe in detail the taping method which I now use for my own stretching program.

TWO-LAYER TAPE RING METHOD:

1. Locate and mark the exact position on the shaft skin of the penis where the tape ring is to be applied when the skin is stretched snugly up over the glans and the extension cone (or other such object).

2. At that location, loosely apply a SINGLE LAYER of $1/2$-inch tape around the shaft of the penis, overlapping the ends of the tape approximately $3/4$ inch. Properly applied, this first layer of tape forms a very loose-fitting ring around the shaft of the penis.

CAUTION: Be sure the extension cone has a large enough diameter to allow the skin and the ring itself to easily slide back and forth over the glans *and to comfortably accommodate a full erection.*

3. Place the extension cone (or other object) over the glans and gently roll or pull the skin up and over the glans and

the cone until the skin is stretched snugly and the tape ring is in the proper position in front of the tip of the cone.

4. With a second piece of tape approximately six or seven inches long, apply two or three additional layers directly on the first tape — wrapped around tightly enough to pucker the first ring so as to hold the cone and the skin in place.

The result is a smaller outer tape ring applied directly to the larger tape ring which is applied to the skin. This "two-layer" tape ring allows the removal of the outer tape (and the cone) as often as needed for urinating and bathing, while allowing the first layer of tape to remain in place on the skin as long as you wish.

Suggestions and discoveries:

1. Having tried no less than six different brands and types of tape, I find that Durapore by 3M holds better on my skin than any other brand I've tried. Also, being made of cloth, it is strong but has soft edges when trimmed to various widths.

2. By measuring the circumference of the shaft of the erect penis, one can find the exact length that the first tape (applied to the skin) must be to insure that the larger ring will accommodate an erection and allow easy insertion of the cone. Measuring, marking, and cutting the tape to the right measurement greatly facilitates the application of the first tape ring.

3. Trim the width of the second tape (the top layers) so that it's slightly narrower than the bottom layer — about a quarter or a third of an inch is ideal. This way, the second layer will not touch the skin at any point; thus, removal is very comfortable. Turn a small tab at the end of this tape to facilitate faster removal. This outer tape can be reused a number of times before it needs to be replaced.

4. Use a hair dryer to dry the first layer of tape immediately after bathing. This allows the tape to remain in place on the skin for a number of days if desired.

5. When I started this taping method, I applied the first layer of tape in the same location on the shaft of the penis each time I replaced it. That location, however, soon became irritated and sore, even using hypoallergenic surgical tape.

At present, I rotate three sets of cones which correspond to three different positions for the first layer of tape on the shaft of the penis. After application, I leave the tape in place for three or four days so that each location has at least six days' rest before tape is reapplied to it. This rotation system keeps my skin relatively free of irritation. I wear a cone in place for 20 to 23 hours — every day.

6. When I first began to use extension cones, I used a 5cm cone during the day and no cone at night. Next, I used a 6.5cm cone during the day and the 5cm cone at night, and so on.

At present, I use three sets of cones of the following lengths:
- Tape in position #1 (nearest the body): 10.0cm in the day, 8.5cm at night.
- Tape in position #2 (mid-position): 9.0cm in the day, 7.5cm at night.
- Tape in position #3 (nearest the glans): 8.0cm in the day, 6.5cm at night.

7. Foam rubber comes in varying degrees of firmness, and I looked at several upholstery shops before I found foam firm enough for my purpose. The firmest foam I could find, however, compresses somewhat when the cone is inserted and taped in place. Therefore, the cone lengths reported above do not accurately reflect the amount of skin that has been gained to date.

8. I sculpt the chamber end of the cone to fit over the entire glans. The outer end is solid foam tip which extends beyond the glans according to the desired extension. I measure the cones from the outer rim of the chamber to the tip. Each cone takes approximately sixty to ninety minutes to make. I don't apply any coating, since these cones are removed before urinating.

9. I wash each set of cones in warm water and mild soap after each rotation and allow them to air-dry for at least 24 hours.

Advantages of this method:

1. The first layer of tape can be removed from the skin by whatever method (soaking, etc.) you prefer, and in whatever

time frame is appropriate for your tolerance.

2. The outer tape and cone can be quickly and painlessly removed as often as necessary for both urinating and bathing, which greatly facilitates hygiene.

3. A satisfactory extension can be achieved with a relatively softer foam since these cones are not hollowed out for urination purposes.

4. Since the foam itself traps air and the cones are not coated with sealer, the glans and inner skin remain comfortably dry. After six months, I have had no problem with either irritation or breaking out from the cones.

Disadvantages of the method:

1. One must remove the outer tape and cone each time for urinating and bathing which means that, away from home, stall toilets must be used.

2. One must replace the cone and outer tape each time after urinating, which is a real nuisance. I have become, however, quite skilled at popping the cone right back in place and replacing the tape in a matter of a few seconds.

3. By keeping the glans area quite dry and with the cones fitting as they do between the glans and the "foreskin," the glans has again lost some of the sensitivity it had gained during the earlier stages of stretching when the glans was covered directly by skin. I have every reason to believe, however, once the use of the cones is discontinued and the glans and foreskin are in permanent contact, that the glans will once again become more moist and more sensitive.

All in all, this two-layer tape ring method has meant the difference between continuing my stretching program and having to abandon it after fifteen months. At present (twenty-two months), I can cover approximately half of the glans when flaccid and can stretch the skin to cover almost the entire glans while erect. Some of the covering during erection is due to an increased mobility of the skin along the entire penile shaft, as well as to additional skin. It will take at least two or three years to gain full and natural-looking coverage of the glans.

Soon to Be Uncircumcised

Dear Soon,

Thanks for your easy-to-follow, do-it-yourself instructions.

For additional information about foreskin restoration, I suggest the excellent book, *The Joy of Uncircumcising!* by Jim Bigelow, Ph.D. (Aptos, California: Hourglass Publishing, 1992).

●◇ ◇●

Dear Bud,

I read about the USA in the Australian newspaper *Campaign*, and have subsequently received your newsletters. I've been reading them time and time again. At last someone has done something about the most shameful practice of all times. Do you realize that for fourteen years I have been living with the "Great Australian Circumcision Nightmare" in real agony and isolation. I immigrated here from Greece as a teenager. In my home country men have always worn their foreskin with pride. The idea of circumcision is considered utterly barbaric, cruel, and inhuman.

In Australia, at least in my generation, it seems that 90 percent of the male population is circumcised. The remaining 10 percent are first- or second-generation immigrants from Europe or Asia. It's hard to understand why most English-speaking people would rather have their men with permanently exposed, hardened, semisensitive glans and carrying a two- to three-inch-wide discolored shaft skin topped by the inevitable dark circumcision ring. In actual fact, they prefer to have their men carry mutilated penises, just as do the so-called primitive aborigines whose "barbaric" circumcision practices they scorn.

Greek Lover

Dear Greek,

To support your contention about the aborigines of Australia, I shall quote a passage from Peter Deeley's recent article "Double Jeopardy Cases" (published in the *Observer*):

"In a remote country town of Australia recently, 28-year-old Aboriginal twins were ritually circumcised by the elders of their tribe with an old pocket knife heated over an open coal fire. The twins, who had left the tribe, had been captured after a chase and forced to undergo the brutal initiation ceremony. Technically, under 'White Man's Law', the elders were committing assault against the brothers."

But the elders were not prosecuted.

It's as if we're back with the "fire" circumcisers. But we can take heart from more recent news. According to a poll of Australian hospitals, the neonatal circumcision rate has fallen drastically in your chosen country. From a high of 90 percent in 1944, the rate of circumcisions being performed in 1980 by state is:

Victoria	28%
New South Wales	42%
Queensland	51%
Tasmania	43%
Western Australia	38%

While we're at it, let's review the latest statistics from another English-speaking nation: Canada. Here are the percentages by province of neonatally circumcised boys in 1984:

Newfoundland	0.4%
Prince Edward Island	40.7%
New Brunswick	12.8% (1983)
Nova Scotia	8.5%
Quebec	6.4%
Ontario	47.0%
Manitoba	35.0% (1983)
Saskatchewan	39.3%
Alberta	44.2% (1983)
British Columbia	18.5%
Yukon Territory	20.1%
Northwest Territories	10.3%

Considering that just a decade earlier the circumcision rate was 60 percent in Ontario and 68 percent in Prince Edward Island, Canadian pelt seems to be making a big comeback.

Now let's take a look at the foreskins of modern India, which is where the English-speaking countries were first introduced to the practice of circumcision. The Moslem

Moguls, who were credited for making the clipcock famous in England, have long since passed into history. Today, the large Moslem minority in India and the men of neighboring Pakistan and Bangladesh are circumcised. But the bulk of the huge population on the Indian subcontinent are uncircumcised and, according to some anthropologists, the Hindu foreskin is the longest on Earth. Of course, the Fakirs in Calcutta, who as a penance drag rocks tied by rope to their elongated foreskins, help perpetuate the Hindu reputation.

The Hindu foreskin survived centuries of religious persecution at the hands of the Moguls. According to historian Allen Edwardes, the Moslem rulers imposed a tax on all uncircumcised travelers in India. Village gates were patrolled by guards who inspected each passing penis, and would not allow an uncircumcised visitor to enter until he paid the tax. Many Hindu merchants, rather than pay the tax, submitted to circumcision. The lower caste Hindu simply stayed home, never to roam and never to sacrifice his foreskin.

While we're snooping around the foreskins of Asia, let's take a trivia break. The Moslem nations are circumcised while the Buddhist are not. The Chinese have the shortest foreskins on Earth, the Thais the most available, and the Japanese the most invisible. (The Japanese of the old tradition considered it immature for a man to appear at a public bath with his foreskin forward. A retracted foreskin was the sign of respect.) The Filipinos in many areas circumcise boys at puberty during family festivals, but do not completely remove the foreskin. Instead they allow it to hang in a lump under the penis to act as a "French Tickler" for the women. Some Philippine islanders do not practice any form of circumcision, while affluent Manilans emulate the Americans with neonatal circumcision.

●◇ ◇●

Dear Bud,

I am a 30-year-old engineer, recently married, living in India, and I am a Hindu. Recently while my ship was on your West Coast I happened to come across your literature. Reading about the Acorn Society got me excited because it reminded me of my own fascination with circumcision and my own eventual circumcision. I was not circumcised at birth because Hindu males are never circumcised. In fact, in my country with its varied religions and customs and rituals, the sole means of identifying a male Hindu is his uncircumcised penis. As you might have read, we have religious riots here every year and rival mobs sometimes strip their victims to identify their religion.

In my case I didn't know such a thing as circumcision existed until my thirteenth year in school. I made friends with two Moslem boys at my boarding school and while showering I became fascinated by their penises. I asked why they were different and they got aroused as they related how they had been circumcised by a barber just a few years prior, when they were eight years old. The results were very successful as I admired the looks of their smooth glans and that bunch of skin which rested in a ringlike formation just behind their coronas. I have never had homosexual urges but their penises turned me on. I became obsessed with looking at circumcised penises because they seemed so beautiful and cute to me. In my country, where 90 percent of the population is poor, seeing naked men and boys is no problem.

I soon laid my hands on as many books as possible to gain a better insight into circumcision: its rituals, methods, and pros and cons. By my twenties I was well schooled in the subject and was thoroughly converted. I wanted to get circumcised. I mentioned my interest to my family and my mother immediately dissuaded me. In my twenty-fourth year and final term at college, I went to a government hospital and had myself circumcised. After a week the bandage was removed and I saw that my circumcision was crudely done and not complete. I regretted going to a medical doctor instead of a Moslem barber.

In my recent years of world travel, I have been to practically all countries of the world and observed hundreds of penises from every race. I have seen the results of various circumcision methods, but only in the United States do I see penises which have been entirely stripped of the frenulum, causing the skin of the shaft to be so nice and tight that the whole appearance of the penis is one of beauty. There is interest in the American penis worldwide and I think it is because of the style. I wistfully long to come to your country one day and have my own penis recircumcised in your best style. This is the reason I am writing to your exclusive Acorn club.

Admirer

Dear Bud,

I think the Acorn club had a predecessor here in Seattle. It was in the skid-row section of town and was advertised as a "sex museum" for men. I was in college when I got up enough nerve to go to the place, and I was wide-eyed and awestruck.

The proprietor was a quack who cured "lost manhood" and all those Victorian problems young men were supposed to have in those rather innocent days. The museum was filled with wax figures much like those in today's museums, but the figures all had chancres and sores on the penises and warts on the pussies. The old man narrated to me, probably thinking he was educating a young morsel on the evils of sex. Then he led me to two huge, perfect representations of penises; one circumcised, the other uncircumcised. He pointed out the differences and then proceeded to give me a long lecture on why all men should be circumcised.

He led me into a back workroom and pointed to a shelf full of jars. He told me the jars were stuffed full of foreskins he had cut off visitors to his museum. He took down a jar and allowed me to examine the contents. I was very impressed. He said the young men he circumcised were cured of all their sexual problems and were good husbands and fathers. Then he took down a jar which was only half-filled and said he would be very happy to add my foreskin to the jar that afternoon. I told him I had to think about it. He wouldn't take no for an answer and gave me a list of fourteen reasons for circumcision and some crude before-and-after cock photos. My poor, bewildered penis was straining in my pants. Then the doorbell rang.

I sat down and studied the list and photos and could hardly restrain myself from pulling out my boner. I could hear the man giving a visitor the same lecture, and then the door to the room opened. In walked a young sailor who appeared as wide-eyed as myself at what he was seeing. I can clearly recall his amazed expression as he was shown the jars of foreskins. "Yes!" the sailor blurted out, "I want a circumcised penis just like that wax one out there." The proprietor turned to me and asked, "And you young man?" "Yes!" I shouted.

As the sailor and I began removing our clothes as instructed, I got scared. In those days I was just not used to being naked in public. Besides, I had an erection a mile long and was embarrassed by it. So, while the sailor was stepping out his skivvies, I put my clothes back on. The museum proprietor was understanding and said, "Well, think about it and come back in a few days." As I was led to the door I couldn't resist a quick glance back at the sailor. He was standing there stark naked and in front of him was the stiffest dick I had ever seen.

Needless to say, the experience left a huge impression on me although I never returned to get my promised circumcision. A few years later I returned to the site only to find out that the museum had been closed by the city health officials. Disappointed, I felt deprived of my circumcision experience. My mind had been set for a circumcision. I went to a medical doctor but he told me I had no reason to be circumcised and refused to do it. I was shattered. Now, after all these years, the Acorn Society comes along. My still-uncircumcised penis will be fully erect when I attend the club's festivities.

All Attention

●◇ ◇●

Dear Bud,

I just heard about the Acorn club, which does circumcisions. I am a baseball player and the fellows call me Pointer. Our fans think I got that name because I'm supposed to have the habit of pointing at the fly ball for the outfielder. What they don't know is that I got the name because of my uncut dick. I've got a real pointing foreskin and I get ribbed about it in the locker room. A couple of the fellows offered to pass the hat to pay for my circumcision. It was supposed to be a joke, but I know damned well they would like to watch while my point gets blunted. I have in truth always wanted to get circumcised and am thinking it might be fun to make a party out of it. Do the Acorn fellows allow guests? I'd like the whole team to be there in uniform and I want to be circumcised wearing my baseball cap. How's that for a send-off?

Ready to Play Ball

Dear Acorn People,

Have fun, fellows. Most of my readers would prefer that I talk you out of joining Acorn. Another foreskin down the drain doesn't exactly make me happy. However, since my argument in the circumcision debate is that infants are not allowed a choice in the matter, how can I criticize you when you do make a choice? What an adult does with his penis is nobody's damned business.

Dear Bud,

I have made a lifelong study of Native Americans and their history, but I have found nothing regarding their circumcision practices. Can you enlighten me on that subject?

Student

Dear Native American Student,

Our colonial forefathers didn't entirely overlook the cocks of the Indians; they duly noted the circumcised penises of the Algonquin tribe of northern New York and named the tribe "the Lost Tribes of Israel." I am not aware of any other North American tribe that practiced routine circumcision.

Indian lore has been full of the love and affection among groups of young warrior braves. Supposedly, some such groups were bonded by group circumcision, becoming blood brothers forever. However, such lore can't be verified. The early Spanish did return to Europe with stories of circumcision among the Aztecs. Mythologist Joseph Campbell in his monumental book *The Mythical Image* told of a strange form of circumcision practiced during the Aztec sacrificial rite. Frenzied men offered their penises to sacrifice and the priest merely sliced a vertical slit on the top of the foreskin. The rite being an annual occurrence, the Aztec foreskins yearly received an additional slit. After a few years of "sacrifice," the foreskins were shredded.

Today, the only routine circumcision of which I am aware among "South of the Border" Americans occurs among the affluent around Mexico City. It is perpetrated as being hygienic, but a remark that a USA member overheard from a circumcised young Mexican ("I am one of the new breed"), makes it sound more like fashion. However, once away from the sprawling Mexican metropolis, Mexico is a sea of foreskin, as is all of Latin America.

Modern American Indians haven't had an easy time holding onto their foreskins. One man wrote to the USA:

> I am a Cherokee Indian in the Army. They told me I had a torpedo-type penis which had to be circumcised. I went to my chaplain, who reminded the medics that the military had agreed to stop circumcising our people. We have special rituals in which the foreskin plays an important role. I wear a bone ring under my skin which was handed down to me from my great-great-grandfather.

Columnist Jack Anderson, in a *Washington Post* article during the seventies titled "Injustice to Indians," wrote:

> There appears to be no end to the injustice inflicted on our neglected native Americans. Documents in our possession describe severe overcrowding, inadequate care and outright malpractice in our Indian Health Service hospitals.
>
> The documents show [nurses] have been taught to perform circumcisions. The documents show that they have performed circumcisions in violation not only of the state's laws but the Health, Education and Welfare Dept.'s rules for protecting human subjects. Moreover, Indian parents weren't told that nurses were circumcising their babies. Claremont's [Oklahoma's Claremont Indian Hospital] chief of pediatrics, Dr. Edwin Jones, who has resigned under fire, said he believed the parents would develop "unnecessary anxiety" if they knew nurses were performing the surgery on their babies.

Dear Bud,

I visited Russia several years ago and met a young man one night in a Leningrad park. He invited me to his apartment and after hiking through the darkened city, we finally came upon his huge apartment block. We stepped over his relatives sleeping on the floor in the small apartment and found privacy inside a closet. He took one look at my circumcised penis and said, *nyet*. I don't think he ever before looked at a cut cock. Aren't there any circumcised men in the Soviet?

Soviet Visitor

Dear Soviet Visitor,

Perestroika, the dissolution of the Soviet Union, and the renaming of St. Petersburg might have changed things in Russia since your visit, but I doubt that your circumcised penis would receive a better reception there today. While Russia supposedly has a 10 percent circumcision rate, the operation is performed only when medically necessary, mostly because of phimosis. The Russians, until recently, have known no other reason to circumcise. To your nocturnal liaison in the Leningrad park you might as well have had an amputated arm.

The old Soviet government, officially atheistic, outlawed religious circumcision. Anyone performing the religious rite of circumcision was subject to arrest. As a result, few Jewish men in the Soviet Union were circumcised. Ironically, however, the huge numbers of Moslem men living in the southern tier of Soviet Republics were circumcised without official interference. The Soviets seemingly considered the Islamic custom of circumcising teenage boys to be a cultural practice rather than a religious one.

Two recent twists remain in the Russian circumcision story. One concerns rumors that many young Russian soldiers held prisoner in Afghanistan chose "conversion" over death. The other is a rumor that the KGB circumcised its recruits who were chosen to be spies in North America. I suppose they learned their lesson when one of their agents quite literally got caught with his foreskin down. Mark Beaumont told the story of "The Spy Who Wasn't Circumcised" a few years ago in *Foreskin Quarterly*. The spy was Conon Molody, who had been born in Russia and brought to the United States by his aunt in the 1930s. When he later became a spy for Russia, he assumed the identity of "Gordon Lonsdale," a Canadian-born Finnish boy who was taken to

Europe by his mother and vanished during WWII. But when Londsdale fell under suspicion, authorities checked out his background. They found that Gordon Lonsdale had been circumcised in infancy by a Dr. Mitchell. "Lonsdale" the suspect was uncircumcised. They arrested him.

●◇　◇●

Dear Bud,

I was visiting my gay neighbor recently and he gave me some of your literature to read. Even though I'm not gay, my dick stood on bone while reading. Well, we relaxed over a beer and discussed the differences between cut and uncut cocks. The subject got me even hotter. With my goddamned dick stretching my trousers out of shape, my neighbor asked me to pull it out because he wanted to try an experiment. He explained that you had written something about the "meat roll" of uncut cocks. I was willing to play, since I was sitting there with a stiff pole between my legs, and I said, "He's all yours." Well, he placed my hard-on between his flat-out palms and commenced to roll my dick between them. Whoa man! My bone got so hard I thought I was turning queer. He rolled my dick for a good hour and my cock stood rigid the entire time. It felt sensational with my cock spinning inside its foreskin. The skin was spinning faster than the rod. Maybe it was because my neighbor was a bodybuilder, and with his great biceps he was able to really tenderize my sausage. He gave up with exhaustion and didn't bring me off, so with just three long strokes I popped off. No one had ever seen me pop my nuts before, but this guy was gay. I could never do it in front of a straight fellow.

I can't wait to get my dick rolled again. My problem is that I dig chicks and I could never ask a woman to roll my cock. She would think I was weird. I wouldn't mind getting it rolled again by a gay fellow but, Mr. Berkeley, with the health crisis thing coming down, do you think it's safe? Just in case you approve and have a guy in mind who has strong hands and good biceps to back them up, I am 21, blond with blue eyes, five-feet-ten with a 30-inch waist, 155 lbs., and my dick is pretty long and my foreskin overhangs while I am on bone. I need the damned thing "meat-rolled" again.

Meat Rolled

Dear Meat Rolled,

Yummm! Oh, pardon me ... what was your question? Is rolling the dick safe sex? It certainly seems to be safe enough, although in your case it might add up to torture for your partner. As long as it's understood that only hands "backed up by strong biceps" are going to touch your sausage, it's safe for everyone. The USA keeps repeating that the visual aspect of sex is an important ingredient in keeping safe sex a satisfying experience.

Meat, I might get lynched by some of my readers for what I am about to suggest, but I think you're limiting yourself unnecessarily. I'm not sure a woman wouldn't enjoy rolling your penis in her hands, too. Inventive foreplay is half the fun of sex and if the "meat roll" gets you as hot as you say it does, I'll bet any partner would find their efforts well rewarded.

•◇ ◇•

Dear Bud,

My biggest problem being uncircumcised is that I can't keep a condom on my penis. I have the long, loose type foreskin and condoms simply get pushed off my dick. I have no trouble stretching a new rubber over my cock, either with the foreskin forward or skinned back, but once I start pumping the condom pushes up my shaft with the motion of the skin. It often ends up in a bunched-up wad under my foreskin and it's very uncomfortable. Besides, I hate to think what it's doing to my partner. It certainly isn't giving us the necessary protection. Do other uncut men report this problem?

Losing My Condom

Dear Condom,

Yes, some uncut men report your problem with condoms, especially those with the long, loose foreskin you describe. There are many sexual acts that are safe and don't require condoms, but penetration is safe only with a rubber. You may want to try Stubs, a cap-type condom that covers only the cockhead on an uncircumcised man. This allows the foreskin to move uninhibitedly over the entire range of the cock. Unfortunately, some men find that these slip off as easily. You'll have to experiment to see how they work for you. If you can't be sure a condom is going to stay on, then it's not going to be safe to use. (If you cannot find Stubs, or a similar product, ask your merchant to order it. There probably aren't enough foreskins out there for merchants to order a large supply.) There's also a small possibility that the man wearing a Stubs could become infected through abrasions on the uncovered part of his penis. This certainly isn't a common route of HIV infection, but based on what we know right now, it can't be ruled out entirely.

There is a wide range of safe-sex activities that do not require rubbers. Check with your counselor, or doctor, or try one of the safe-sex seminars offered by AIDS groups and educators. I think you'll find some techniques that you can safely enjoy. In any case, please be honest about your HIV status.

●◇ ◇●

Dear Bud,

J/O rules in my house. With the coming of the AIDS epidemic, I have turned to masturbation almost exclusively. I can pound my long 10-inch uncircumcised penis for hours. I love to watch my long foreskin roll up and down in its hypnotic rhythm, making an audible "snap" as it closes its tip over the glans to once again smooth itself out over the throbbing shaft. With my dick as my gear shift, I can enter wondrous worlds of fantasy and beauty. It's like entering a new dimension: an inner dimension that takes me out of the mundane world. I have found that the most satisfying sexual experience is to share these fantasies with a J/O buddy, while we both pump on our dicks. It is safe sex at its best.

J/O Lover

Dear J/O,

In this age of AIDS, most sex counselors advise masturbation. It's quite a far cry from the Victorian anti-masturbation hysteria of a century ago! Today, masturbation is considered to be healthy. It can reduce stress and keep the body's systems lubricated. The USA promotes J/O over less-safe practices by emphasizing the visual component of sexual arousal. The penis is beautiful, cut or uncut. Watching a man's penis being masturbated can be breathtakingly exciting. Why hide it? And now that J/O is in, what could be more fitting to have nature's "pumper" — the foreskin — in fashion at the same time?

●◇ ◇●

Dear Bud,

I sent your material about neonatal circumcision to my family in Texas. I have four brothers down there, all uncut, and they're producing boys like crazy. I just wanted to remind them of our family tradition. We keep our menfolk whole. I had heard a couple of my sisters-in-law had different ideas for their sons. Well, from last report, the family is repopulating the state of Texas with foreskin. Yippee!

Your Buddy

Howdy Buddy,

Yeaaa! Hey, pardner, aren't we damned lucky? To be Americans, that is. After my criticisms of forced circumcision, our mechanical society, and so on, I still have to admit several things about our country. First, where else on Earth could we write so freely and speak up so loudly about our cocks? Second, where else could a club like the USA exist? This place is great and it's full of enthusiastic, thoughtful dudes like you. Tex, keep it up!

In honor of your Texan brood, let's sing the anthem written for us by a Canadian member of the Uncircumcised Society of America. It is to be sung to the tune of "America the Beautiful":

> O hood divine, O skin sublime
> O foreskin dark or fair
> O wrinkled tip, O pouting lip
> Your beauty is all there.
> Unveil, unveil man's tool of life
> and cover it again...
> The thrills are true, the pleasure too;
> Why can't all men own you?

●◇ ◇●

Dear Bud,

I think the potential scope of the USA is far broader than "gay" or "circumcision." It has elements of a potent male liberation movement. Male liberation, as we have seen it so far, is a phony. It merely buries us deeper into our matriarchal society. Men learning how to cry? What a stupid issue. Men have always cried. Most of us have no hang-ups about crying. Our hang-ups are with our penises. We should be proud of them, free to talk about them, free to enjoy them without guilt. We are men because we have cocks. Our male libidos belong in our cocks. Instead, our society has transplanted our libidos from our penis to our fists and the guns in our hands.

Our penises are looked upon with disgust and derision, while our National Sentinel proudly holds a rifle. This "loaded gun" culture of ours is the fault of our history of militarism. Through countless generations of war and struggle, men have become expendable to society and women become widows. Women, constantly prepared for widowhood, protect themselves from "the men" through the controls of myths, old wives' tales, traditions, and taboos. The matriarchal pantheon is defended by the sons who are marched off to war. Why not amputate their foreskins, desensitize them, deodorize them to please the matriarchy?

How can men enjoy the full meaning of manhood in a society which can't stand to look at us straight in our balls? Why shouldn't men have the right to "cock-talk"? It has nothing whatever to do with gay, straight, or bi. It has everything to do with the healthy male libido being squarely where it belongs: in the penis. The violence of the fist and the gun is destroying our world. The gun between the legs would give only love and life to mankind ... and a future. USA, you've got a big job to do.

My Gun's between My Legs

Dear Legs,

Wow! You've given the USA a tall order. First, we don't mean to associate sexual orientation with the question of circumcision. Their only connection can be Thomas Szasz's contention (in *The Manufacture of Madness*) that "there is no significant difference between the former persecution of masturbators and the present persecution of homosexuals."

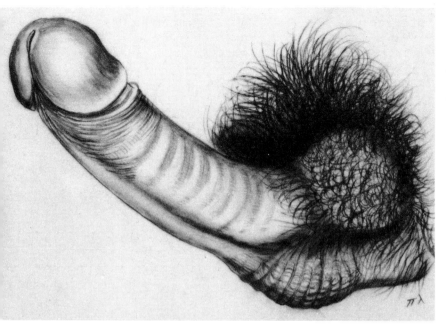

A natural penis with a normal foreskin pulled back in fullest rigid erection at about a 140-degree angle. Plateau phase of arousal, with testicles drawn completely up above the shaft just before orgasm, leaving scrotum completely empty.

Second, I am not sure whether our "loaded gun" culture is the result of a matriarchy, or a patriarchy, or both, or neither. The women's liberation groups blame the patriarchy. But labels are not important. The USA must take one step at a time and our first step is to demand the right of choice for men. Each man should have his own "informed" choice about which style of penis he prefers for himself. Whether he chooses to be circumcised or uncircumcised is not our business. His right to choose is our business. But, like the bewildered boy staring at the wax models of penises in the museum, how do you make such a choice? We have heard from advocates of both circumcised and uncircumcised penises. Which will it be? The sleek all-American clipcock (of worldwide renown) or the pillcock with its pumper?

Today, more American men can make that choice for themselves than could do so a generation ago. In another generation, I hope we will recognize this as a choice that every man should have as his birthright.